THE BODY
HAS ITS REASONS

THE BODY HAS ITS REASONS

Self Awareness Through Conscious Movement

*Thérèse Bertherat
and Carol Bernstein*

HEALING ARTS PRESS
Rochester, Vermont

To Mme. A., a well-known lawyer who confuses her self-image with her professional image and is afraid she'll lose her authority if she loses the stiffness in her neck and the aggressive expression on her face.

To Admiral B., who, feeling on the decline at retirement age, learned how to breathe, to hold his head (rather than his jaw) high—and grew an inch and a half taller.

To Mlle. C., who had her nose, her chin, her eyelids, and her breasts redone, but sheds genuine tears because no one can redo her life.

To D., who takes his body to be treated as he takes his car to be repaired: "Do whatever needs to be done. I don't want to know about it." But I have nothing to tell him that deep down he doesn't already know.

To Mlle. E., virgin and martyr, who for forty years has been claiming she wants to get rid of her stomach, which bulges like that of a woman eight months pregnant. Always smiling and seemingly cooperative, she refuses to make the changes that would deliver her.

To Mme. F., who hates her body, claims to adore people who don't resemble her, yet seeks only to humiliate them.

To G., who as a teen-ager closed her eyes so successfully to herself that she managed to sleep sixteen hours out of twenty-four. Her shoulders drooping, the back of her neck hollow, her head flung back, she glided through life like a sleepwalker until one day, in a mirror, she met up with an aging woman, eyes wide open in disbelief.

For the Comte de H., who regards his health as "an affair of state," refusing to admit he's sick unless the National Health Insurance Plan covers the illness.

Healing Arts Press
One Park Street
Rochester, Vermont 05767

Note to the reader: *This book is intended as an informational guide. The remedies, approaches, and techniques described herein are meant to supplement, and not to be a substitute for, professional medical care or treatment. They should not be used to treat a serious ailment without prior consultation with a qualified healthcare professional.*

LIBRARY OF CONGRESS CATALOGING-IN-PUBLICATION DATA
Bertherat, Thérèse.
        The body has its reasons.

        Translation of: Le corps a ses raisons.
        Reprint. First American ed. published: New York: Pantheon Books, c1977.
        Bibliography: p.
        1. Mind and body. 2. Self-perception. 3. Exercise therapy.
    4. Self-actualization (Psychology) I. Berstein, Carol. II. Title
    BF162.B3813 1989   613   89-2059
    ISBN 0-89281-298-2

Printed and bound in the United States

10 9 8 7 6 5 4 3 2

Healing Arts Press is a division of Inner Traditions International

Distributed to the book trade in Canada by Publishers Group West (PGW),
    Toronto, Ontario

Distributed to the health food trade in Canada by Alive Books, Toronto and
    Vancouver

Distributed to the book trade in the United Kingdom by Deep Books, London

Distributed to the book trade in Australia by Millennium Books, Newtown, N.S.W.

Distributed to the book trade in New Zealand by Tandem Press, Auckland

Distributed to the book trade in Europe by HDG Distrirep, The Netherlands

Distributed to the book trade in South Africa by Alternative Books, Randburg

Contents

Introduction

Your Body, That House You Don't Live In

Exactly where you are at this very moment, there is a house that bears your name. You're its sole owner but, a very long time ago, you lost the keys. So you stay outside; you're familiar only with the façade. You don't live in it. That house, the hideaway of your most deeply buried, repressed memories, is your body.

"If walls could hear . . ." In the house of your body, they can. The walls which have heard everything and never forgotten anything are your muscles. In the stiffness and the tension, in the pains and deficiencies of the muscles of your back, your neck, your legs, your arms, your diaphragm, your heart, and also of your face and your sexual organs, your complete history is revealed, from your birth to the present day.

Without even realizing it, from the first months of your life you have reacted to family, social, and moral pressures. "Stand like this, like that. Don't touch things. Don't touch yourself. Be nice. Defend yourself. Hurry up. Don't run . . ." Confused, you bent your will and your body as much as you could. To conform, you deformed yourself. In the place of your real body, naturally harmonious and dynamic, a foreign body has been substituted. You have trouble accepting it. In your innermost self, you reject it.

That's life, you say, you can't do anything about it. I say that you can, and that you alone can do something. It's not too late. It's never too late to free yourself from the programming of your past, to assume your responsibility for your body, to discover possibilities you don't even suspect.

To be is never to cease being born. But how many of us allow ourselves to die a little every day, incorporating ourselves so successfully into the structures of contemporary living that we lose our lives because we lose sight of ourselves?

We leave to doctors, psychiatrists, architects, politicians, employers, our husbands, our lovers, our children the responsibility for our health, our well-being, our security, our pleasures. We entrust our lives, our bodies, to others, sometimes to those who haven't asked for this responsibility and find themselves burdened by it, and frequently to those who are part of the institutions whose primary objective is to reassure us, and in that way to repress us. (And how many people of every age are there whose bodies still belong to their parents? Obedient children, they wait in vain all their lives for permission to live. Psychological minors, they are the uncomprehending spectators of other people's lives, although they often, in their ignorance, become the strictest censors.)

By giving up our autonomy we abdicate our individual sovereignty. We belong to the powers, to the individuals who have claimed us. If we demand our liberty so emphatically, it's because we feel that we are slaves; and the most lucid of us acknowledge that we are slave-accomplices. But how could we be anything else since we aren't even masters of our first house, the house of our body?

And yet it is possible for you to find the keys to your body again, to take possession of it, to live in it at last, and to find your proper vitality, health, and autonomy.

But how? Certainly not by regarding your body as a necessarily defective machine that encumbers you, as a machine made up of isolated parts, each of which (head, back, feet, nerves) must be entrusted to a specialist whose authority and verdict you blindly accept. Certainly not by being content to label yourself once and for all "nervous," "insomniac," "constipated," or "frail." And certainly not by trying to fortify yourself through exercises, which are no more than the forced drilling of the body considered as a piece of meat, as unintelligent, as an animal to be disciplined.

Our body is ourself. We are what we appear to be. The way we appear is the way we are. But we don't want to admit it. We don't dare look at ourselves. We don't even know how to look at ourselves. We confuse the visible with the superficial. We're only interested in what we cannot see. We even go so far as to be contemptuous of the body and of those who are interested in it. Without stopping to understand our form—our body—we rush to interpret our content: our psychological, sociological, historical structures. All our life we juggle words so that they'll reveal the reasons for our behavior. And what if we were to seek, through our sensations, the reasons of our body?

Our body is ourself. It is our only perceptible reality. It is not opposed to our intelligence, to our feelings, to our soul. It includes them and shelters them. By becoming aware of our body we give ourselves access to our entire being—for body and spirit, mental and physical, and even strength and weakness, represent not our duality but our unity.

In this book I'll tell you about the investigations and the natural methods of those who regard the body as an indissoluble whole. I will also recommend some movements which do not belittle or reduce your intelligence but, on the contrary, develop muscular intelligence and require, a priori, the perspicacity of those who practice them.

These movements originate from inside your body; they are not imposed from the outside. There is nothing mystical or mysterious about them. Their goal is not to have you escape from your body, but to avoid having your body continue to escape you, and your life with it.

Until now these movements were defined only by what they are not: exercises, gymnastics. But what word can communicate that an individual's body and his life are the same thing and that he can't live his life fully if, preliminarily, he hasn't been able to awaken the dead zones of his body?

Before writing this book I wasn't particularly concerned with finding an appropriate name for the movements. The results obtained through them were definition enough. If pressed, I would sometimes say that I taught "anti-exercises," or "anti-gymnastics" —always adding that this work could only be understood through the body, through live experience.

But a book is made only of words. So I tried to invent one to sum up the essential character of those movements known only by those who practiced them. A host of Greek and Latin roots were combined in every which way. All the results were partially suitable; none was very satisfactory. And then one day a word that existed already, a very simple word that I used quite often, sounded right. Preliminary. Preliminaries. I decided to call the movements that prepare the body—the entire individual—to be able to live fully "Preliminaries."

Throughout this book and listed at the end, you'll find descriptions of Preliminaries through which you'll come to realize that you can stop wearing yourself out needlessly and stop aging prematurely by using, not ten or a hundred times more energy than necessary as you are now doing, but only the appropriate energy for each gesture.

You can allow yourself to drop your masks, your disguises, your poses, to act no longer "as if" but to be, and to have the courage of your authenticity.

You can find relief from a multitude of ills—insomnia, constipation, digestive problems—as you make muscles that today you're not even sure you have work *for* you and not against you.

You can awaken your five senses, sharpen your perceptions, have and know how to project an image of yourself that satisfies you and that you can respect.

You can affirm your individuality, rediscover your initiative, your confidence in yourself.

You can increase your intelligence by improving your control of the nerve network between your brain and your muscles.

You can unlearn the bad habits that make you favor and thus overdevelop and deform certain muscles, reconsider the unintelligent automatic movements of your body, and discover its efficiency, its spontaneity.

You can become a polyathlete who can always count on the equilibrium, the strength, and the grace of his body.

You can free yourself from problems of frigidity or impotence and, once you have cleared the obstacles set up over the years by your body, you can have the rare satisfaction not only of living there fully yourself but of sharing your "living space" with someone else.

No matter what your age, you can open the traps that have imprisoned your inner life and your body's behavior and reveal the free, beautiful, well-made individual that you were meant to be.

If I speak to you with so much conviction and enthusiasm, it's because I see these wagers won every day. In this book, I'm only going to talk about what has really been experienced by me, by my students, and by others who began to assume their lives when they started to live in their bodies.

I thank my collaborator, who, having neither professional training nor prejudice, but a lot of intuition and a very personal sense of synthesis, helped me to understand that the questions raised by my work were inseparable from those raised by life itself.

Thérèse Bertherat

Paris, April 1975

THE BODY
HAS ITS REASONS

1

The House on
the Dead-End Street

Until that day, I'd lived as a vagabond. There had never been a family home, a place to go back to. I'd married another wanderer, a medical student. Together we'd made the usual tour of furnished rooms and hospital quarters for resident medical students, and now we were entitled to a suburban apartment reserved for public officials, but where we couldn't paint a wall without the administration's permission. In the fall, we planned to move to Paris and settle at last.

More than a desire, living in my own house had become a pressing need. And I knew that for me to be happy in my house I would have to find it myself.

So I went to Paris with a list of streets where there might still be some private houses. A friend had given me the name of a woman—he thought that she gave exercise classes or something like that—who lived on a pleasant mews street in the 14th arrondissement where there were some small houses and artists' studios.

All day long I met people who seemed to boast about having found the last available house in Paris. My feet, my calves were very sore; my neck, my jaw were in knots; my morale was faltering. So I did what I'd grown accustomed to doing when I was displeased with the world and with myself. I bought my favorite women's magazine and, settled down in a comfortable bistro, I leafed through photographs of carefree models in fictitious situations.

There were also several pages of exercises designed to give me my choice of larger breasts, smaller breasts, legs like Dietrich's, buttocks like Bardot's. I flipped through those pages very quickly. The very idea of gymnastics wore me out beforehand and automatically reminded me of noisy, foul-smelling high school gyms. With greater interest, I took a look at the makeup recommended for that week.

When I left the bistro, I bought myself the eye shadow about whose benefits I had just read. I applied it right away, as well as a foundation cream that tanned me instantly. Hidden behind my new face, I decided to go and see Suze L.

There was a linden tree; there was even a peach tree! At the end of this dead-end street with its small, overgrown gardens, I saw a house with closed shutters. Could it be that nobody lived there?

Soft, low, the voice seemed to come from far away. I turned around and found myself face to face with a woman who was still beautiful. I would have expected to find coquettishness in the expression on her face, but there was only generosity.

"Sad-looking today, but beautiful when open."

"Who?"

"Why, the house you're looking at."

"Somebody lives there?"

"Yes."

To hide my disappointment, I couldn't think of anything better than to change the subject.

"Do you know Suze L.?"

The woman smiled slightly.

"Very well. At least, I think so."

"She gives gym classes, doesn't she?" I said, unable to control a slight grimace.

"Yes, it's a kind of gymnastics, but without grimaces." The sound of heels on the cobblestones; she turned around and waved to two young women who were going toward one of the houses.

"A class starts in ten minutes. Do you want to try it?"

All I could think of saying was, "But I don't have the proper clothing."

"I'll lend you some tights," she said and turned away.

So I followed her to a brick house nearly hidden behind trees and bushes.

A large, square room lined with books, paintings, and photographs. On the floor several wicker baskets filled with tennis balls and brightly colored balls. A high stool of pale wood. I found myself with the two young women whom I had just seen, a man whom I took at first for Bourvil,* and a plump, smiling woman who was at least seventy. All in footless tights, they were seated on the floor, looking glad to be there.

As for me, in baggy tights, with a splitting headache and my toes tense and sore, I wasn't glad at all. I wanted to rest, not to do gymnastics. Gymnastics. A word to chew on, a word for the mouth but not for the body. Certainly not for mine. I consoled myself with the thought that Suze L. was not very young any more and that half her students were even older than she. So maybe she wouldn't make us go through too many contortions.

She came in, she too in tights and a full, sand-colored blouse.

"Everything all right?"

Everyone nodded.

She picked up one of the baskets and distributed the balls. She handed me a green one. "Since you like trees," she said with a smile. Then she sat down on her stool.

* Bourvil: a popular French character actor.

"You are going to stand up, feet parallel. Place the ball on the ground. Now roll the ball under your right foot. Imagine that there is ink on the ball and that you want to ink your whole foot—under the toes, under the sole, around the edges. Ink it well. Everywhere. Take your time."

She speaks slowly, softly. Her voice penetrates the silence of the room without breaking it.

"That's it. Now let the ball go and shake the foot that was supporting you. Good. Put your two feet side by side. Very good. Tell me what you feel."

"I feel as though my right foot were sinking into the ground a little bit, as though I were walking on sand," said the elderly lady.

"I feel the toes of my right foot have become wider."

"I have the feeling that my right foot is my real foot and that my left one is made out of wood."

I don't say anything. I'm looking at my feet as though I'd never seen them before. I find the right foot prettier than the left, with its pathetic, squashed-together toes.

"Now lean over without bending your legs and let your arms hang down in front."

I look at my arms. My left hand is four inches from the floor. My right hand touches it!

"You can stand up now."

Everybody stands up.

"Do you know why your right arm goes down lower than your left arm?"

"Because of the ball," says one of the young women.

"Yes. The ball helped you relax the muscles of your foot. And since the body is a whole, all the muscles of your leg and your back have loosened up, too. They no longer act as a brake."

Next she asks us to roll the ball under the left foot. When I bend over, my two hands touch the floor.

"Now you're going to lie flat on your back, your arms close to your body. Where are your body's points of contact with the floor?"

I am balanced on the back of my skull, the tips of my shoulder blades, and my buttocks.

"How many vertebrae are resting on the floor?"

None of my vertebrae are touching the floor. I don't see how they could.

"Bend your knees. You'll be more comfortable."

But what kind of exercise is this that's concerned with my comfort? I thought the more you made the body suffer, the more good you did it.

"Is that better? Is your waist resting on the floor?"

You could have rolled those miniature cars my son plays with through the hollow under my waist.

"Now press the soles of your feet and all your toes firmly on the floor and lift up the lower part of your buttocks a little. Not too much, just enough to be able to pass your fist through. Let yourselves down. Lift up and let yourselves down several times. Gently. Find a rhythm that's suited to you. You're not forgetting to breathe, are you?"

Concentrating on the movement of my pelvis, I had, of course, forgotten.

"All right. Place the lower part of your back on the floor while trying to aim your coccyx toward the ceiling. Is your waist touching the floor now?"

I still have my tunnel. Suze L. rolls toward me a rubber ball, as large and soft as a grapefruit.

"Place the ball at the bottom of your spinal column."

With a furtive gesture, I slide the ball under my behind.

"That's all. Just stay like that and breathe. Put your hands on your ribs so that you can better feel how they move when you breathe. There is no relationship at all, though, between your waist and your jaw. No use clenching it. That's better. Now imagine that you're sinking your finger lightly into your navel.

It's going down toward the floor and your stomach's going with it."

Her voice seems far away, hushed. I feel all alone with my navel.

"Take the ball away. Lay your back down. Lay your entire back down on the floor."

I obey. I feel calm, absorbed; a pleasant warmth spreads throughout my body.

"What about your waist?"

Slowly I slide my hand. The tips of my fingers barely enter the hollow.

"It's coming along," says Suze L., as satisfied as I am. "Now I'm going to ask you to do something which you may not have done for a very long time. Keep your back on the floor. Bend your legs. Stretch your arms out in front of you and grab your toes in your hands."

When my eighteen-month-old daughter does this, I think she's adorable. But when I myself do it, I feel absolutely ridiculous.

"It's funny," says the old lady.

"You have your toes securely in your hands? Now you're going to try to unbend your legs. But don't strain yourself."

My legs unbend a little, very little. I roll from one side to the other. I feel stupid and vulnerable.

"It's not working," says Bourvil's stand-in.

"You'll see," says Suze L. "Sit down. Feel behind your right knee. What do you find?"

"A bone on each side," says one of the young women.

"Those aren't bones. Those are the tendons of your muscles and they can be made more supple. You can do it yourselves. Take hold of them and play with them as though you were jazz musicians and they were strings of a bass violin. Take your time."

I play "Blue Moon" at a slow tempo with no conviction whatsoever.

"All right? Now lie down flat on your back again. Grab the

toes of your right foot. Try to unbend your leg a little, then bend it back again. Then start again. Do that several times without straining yourself. Wait for your body to grant you permission to go further."

My leg unbends a little more each time. But I'm shaky. I roll from one side to the other.

"You roll like that because you're not breathing."

I expel a hearty gust of air from my mouth and make a lot of noise doing it.

"Not through your mouth! The mouth has many pleasant uses, but inhaling and exhaling are not among them. You must always breathe through the nose."

One more theory on the proper way to breathe, I say to myself. Nevertheless, I breathe through my nose. And my body is immediately stabilized!

"Very good. Unbend, bend again, gently. Are you making progress?"

"I've done it!" shouts one of the young women. She's holding on to her toes and her leg is perfectly straight.

"Good. What about the rest of you?"

I unbend. I bend again. I breathe through my nose. I start to discover a certain pleasure that I can't quite account for. And then, there it is. There's my leg straightening out almost completely.

"Very good," says Suze L. "Do you understand what's happened? By making your tendons more supple, by relaxing the back of your leg, you've loosened up your back too, stretched it out. The body is a complete work; you can't know what it's about through selected extracts. Now we'll work on our left side."

We did that with the same results and then we stood up. I was standing as I'd never stood before: my heels sank into the floor, my entire foot, the sole and all the toes were firmly planted. I felt stable, sure of myself.

Then Suze L. had us do several other movements without using balls. My confident body followed the voice that was guiding it. I knew that it was Suze L.'s voice, but it seemed to be coming from inside myself, expressing my body's needs and helping it to satisfy them.

After a little while, Suze L. distributed some balls, about as big as apples. They were fairly heavy, about a pound.

"Place the ball to your right. Lie down on your back again, your arms the length of your body, your fingers stretched out as well. Touch the ball with your fingertips. Push it a little toward your feet, then bring it back a little bit toward the palm of your hand. Make small, slow movements. Push it. Bring it back. As though your arm were elastic."

Her voice floats above our heads like a cloud.

"Now take the ball in your palm. Press your elbow down and lift the ball up. That's it. Let the ball roll gently in your palm and feel when the ball is in equilibrium and you don't have to tighten your arm or your hand. Make your palm into a bed where the ball can rest. Your fingers are no longer touching the ball? Good. Now close your hand over the ball again and place it next to your body and leave your arm close to your body, too. Good."

She's no longer saying anything. No one is saying anything. In the silence, I have a sense of well-being that I haven't known since that summer when, alone in the sea, I floated on my back in clear, motionless water . . . or perhaps sometimes after making love.

"How do you feel?"

"I feel very good," volunteers the man. "I feel relaxed. My shoulder, my arm, my hand have a pleasant weight. I can feel their volume. I feel that I exist in space, that I have three dimensions. Do you see what I mean?"

"I see. And you?"

Suze L. is standing next to me. I tell her: "I feel that my right eye is larger than my left eye and that the right corner of my mouth is relaxed but on the left side I'm grimacing."

"It's more than a feeling. Your right eye is actually larger and your mouth is precisely as you describe it. Marianne, turn around, please, and look at our friend."

"It's crazy," says the young woman. "Her right eye is wide open. The left looks so small, and dull, too."

"Let's not leave our left side in distress like that," says Suze L. And she has us do the same movements on the left side.

"Stand up now and stretch."

My back stretches out completely. There's no end to a back. Nor to an arm, nor to a leg. I had thought I was exhausted when I arrived and now I feel my energy circulating throughout my body. I realize I'm smiling. I look toward the stool because my smile is for Suze L. But she's no longer there. Around me people are starting to get dressed. The class is over.

Once dressed, I look for Suze L., but I can't find her. I go out into the passageway. My feet no longer twist on the cobblestones. My toes take hold of the ground; my gait is elastic. My shoulders are no longer knotted. My neck feels long and supple. My arms sway. Walking, just plain walking, is a pleasure.

Is it my imagination or are the colors of that tree brighter, the contours of the leaves sharper? And all those earth smells, that sultry wind? Could spring have begun while I was in Suze L.'s house?

And my house: the one that I'd come to look for in Paris and thought I hadn't found? What if I had found it? What if the first house of my life was my body?

2

The Fortress

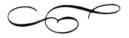

As before when it had wanted to make love, eat, drink, now it was my body that directed me to satisfy its desire for well-being. So each week I took the highway back to that dead-end street that had become an opening toward myself.

In addition to the people from the first class, I found myself with a businessman who seemed to be wearing a tight collar and tie even when dressed in a tee shirt, a forty-year-old woman, radiantly pregnant for the first time, and a grave and absorbed teen-ager who had said her last word—"no"—at the age of five.

Often agitated and fidgety on arrival, we all calmed down during the hour we spent at Suze L.'s. Her serenity called forth our own. In the mirrorless room, she offered us an image of what we could be and to which we were irresistibly drawn.

After the last class of the season, I waited for the others to go. Obviously, I had wanted to tell her something. Something that had seemed important to me. Something that now totally escaped me.

"I wanted to thank you. That's all."

She smiled at me. We shook hands. And I left.

I was in my car before I remembered what I'd wanted to

tell her. I wanted to work. I wanted to try to do work like hers. My husband was very interested by the classes I'd described to him and had advised me to ask Suze L. about the necessary training. He even thought I could work with his patients in his department at the psychiatric hospital. He didn't think of them as "cases," madmen from whom sane people had to protect themselves, but as human beings to be respected for the profound truth they express through their speech and their behavior.

How had I "forgotten" all that?

The long summer vacation. At peace with myself, with my body, I watched my children and my husband playing in the pine forest above Nice and had the feeling that we were the privileged people of the earth, invulnerable.

October 15th. Six o'clock in the morning. Sunday. On the phone a ceremonious voice I don't recognize: "Madame . . . your husband . . . has been wounded . . . a bullet . . . . "

I'm sitting on the edge of the bed still warm from his body. Under the shutters daylight is starting to enter the room. It was still night only a quarter of an hour ago when he was called on emergency duty because a patient was threatening the nurses with a pistol. A quarter of an hour ago it was still yesterday. Yesterday we were making plans with the children for a birthday party: mine.

I'm running through the corridor of a hospital on the outskirts of Paris. I pass a waiting room, an office. I hear only my own steps. I see only my shadow. There is no one here.

Where are they? Where is he? Why did they bring him here? Nowhere. All those hospitals in Paris that are so well equipped, so close by the highway deserted at this hour . . .

At the end of the hall a door opens. A woman in white walks toward me without hurrying.

"I'm Madame Bertherat. Where is he?"

"In the operating room."

I followed her glance toward the staircase: an arrow with the words "operating room" written on it.

"The waiting room is across the hall."

"Hit where?"

"Near the heart."

Sit. In the angle of the first step and the wall. Here it's still night. Here it's yesterday. Nobody is speaking to me. Nobody has spoken yet.

The corridor is deserted again. Then through a small barred window, daylight enters, as though by mistake. But what's done is done. It can't turn back. So it comes forward, but furtively, grazing the wall.

A nurse is coming down the stairs. I press against the wall. Her watch passes in front of my eyes. Eight o'clock. Six o'clock and now eight o'clock. "I'm Madame Bertherat." She continues on her way. Only yesterday at my husband's hospital those words were enough. People smiled at me. Brought me a chair. Today I'm a beggar. I stretch out my hand toward the white uniform that turns around sharply: "Everybody's with him."

A man in a suit suddenly appears in the hall. He jostles me as he runs up the stairs.

"The surgeon," whispers the nurse.

Burning panic shoots through the back of my neck and lodges in my throat. Six o'clock and now eight o'clock. Two hours with a bullet near his heart.

"There was no surgeon here?"

"It's Sunday."

"He hasn't been operated on yet?"

"Of course he has." She's already wasted enough time on me. One last bit of information, out of kindness: "By the intern on duty."

The wall is slimy: it's in a cold sweat.

"You're not going to stay here."

I am going to stay here. Under the arrow. Under the words. I'm in the wall now. Across the hall, daylight keeps moving closer, a dirty green. A hot mug against my fingers. The smell of coffee. In the hall, steps and voices.

"What about that blood type?"

"The lab hasn't called back yet."

I grab a blue lab coat.

"What blood type?"

The woman pulls at her coat. A useless effort. My hand understands now that it alone can tear words out of the silence.

"Your husband's. They took a sample into the city." Into the city. "It's Sunday." It's Sunday. In a hospital. I believed. I had always believed.

Nobody goes by any more. Only time. The day advances along the opposite wall. Someone's running. White shoes brush against me as they climb the stairs. I ask them what's happening. A spontaneous, breathless voice.

"Blood. At last."

"There wasn't any?"

"Wasn't any more. Had to go to Paris for it."

My voice beats against the wall. "Because it's Sunday."

A door opens. Closes.

The day stands up straight. Time stops. Noon. Six o'clock, eight o'clock, the blood hour, and now noon. Behind the wall, a cranking elevator. Its door opens. A stretcher. A sheet. Over a body. It's him. But it's not him. A face I've never seen. Two trails of blood run from his nostrils, congeal on his cheeks. An arm pushes me back. But I hadn't leaned forward.

"Wait. We're going to tidy him up a bit."

A nurse with a flat, jovial, red face. She turns her back to me, leaving behind her the words: "The operation went very well."

Relieved, I stand there motionless, enveloped in the words that explain everything: "The operation went very well." If no doctor, no intern, no nurse, no attendant ever came to talk to me, it's because they were all tired after such a long operation so well performed. And ever since they've been discussing the operation, congratulating one another.

The nurse comes out of a small room at the end of the hall. She goes into another room and closes the door behind her.

He's in a bed now. His feet are sticking out from under the sheet. I cover them. I'm sure he wouldn't like to show his feet here. A chair. I sit down. I can't bring myself to look at his face. My gaze stops at his throat. In which there's a small tube. They've done a tracheotomy! "The operation went very well." The sound of those words in my ear is louder than his noisy breathing.

You can't see the sun through these windows of unpolished glass. But the light has changed. It must be afternoon. The days are short in October. Today must be about four minutes shorter than yesterday. Lose four minutes. Lose only four minutes. His eyes have opened. He's looking at me. I smile. He wants to speak. His lips, his tongue won't obey. "The operation went very well." All we'll need are tenderness and love to get life to circulate again throughout his body.

It's best that none of his colleagues from the hospital have come. We're better off alone together. They must be busy with the police, or simply with their families. It's Sunday. I don't need anyone since "the operation went very well."

A metallic sound. Loud. Deafening. A machine breaking. "The operation went very well." Breathe! Even if breathing should tear his lungs, rip his bandages apart, expose his shattered heart! Breathe!

His hands scratch at his bandages, seem to want to draw them toward him, toward his mouth. *"All dying people do that."*

He told me that himself. "We say that they're 'collecting.' Warmth, I suppose, what's left of their life."

"The operation went very well . . . the operation . . ."

"I was his friend." Was! "I'm B."

Near the door, motionless, a fat man, sloppy and uncombed.

"Call a doctor! A surgeon! Call another surgeon!"

His voice is flat, firm: "That isn't done."

Screaming isn't done either. Striking out with your fists isn't done either. Beating your head against the wall isn't done either. Sitting down is done. Waiting is done. So I sit down and nobody comes to disturb me as I wait for him to die.

When my heart doesn't knock against my ribs any more, isn't lodged in my throat any more, doesn't leap into my mouth any more, doesn't plunge into my guts any more, I know that I have nothing more to wait for.

And I know that there has been a dying to which I was not a witness and a dying to which I was a witness and to which I was an accomplice. And that I will be an accomplice no longer. And that I will be believing and confident no longer.

The fat man moves aside and lets me go by. This time there are people in the corridor. A crowd. Journalists. Who took the time to call them? Who, not having dared to come to the man, had already transformed him into an event? To the journalists' questions, I reply, "The operation went very well," and I go away.

"In the name of the administration . . ."

Standing before his coffin at the Church of Saint-Séverin, I clasp my children's hands in mine as the prefect's words pass over our heads in solemn cadence.

"Today we weep . . ."

The prefect isn't weeping. Nor are we, neither my children nor myself. Not here.

"To the detriment of his family obligations . . ."

What's he talking about? The only "detriment" was that I too abandoned him in that hospital. The "detriment" was not daring to do what isn't done. It was not to have taken him to Paris myself. It was to have let all those hours go by, the hours that were to be the last of his life.

"It is up to you, madame, to tell your young children that their father personified a great . . ."

But you don't know anything about that, Monsieur le Préfet. Your words can't teach me anything. I alone know what it is up to me to do. I alone, in my body, knew what to do. When I went back to the house, the children ran toward me, amazed by my long absence. What about the party? Where's Papa? I answered them with my body. I held them against my stomach, my thighs, my breasts so that all the tenderness, all the security, all the words that emanated in silence from my body could penetrate theirs. "Blow on it," they used to say when they'd hurt themselves. To blow out through all my pores: that, Monsieur le Préfet, is what it was up to me to do.

But the prefect was talking about a citation bestowed by the Order of the Nation. Here at last was a subject he knew something about.

"We'll take the children," said the man on the phone. "You need to rest."

He was a psychiatrist, one of my husband's colleagues, and he too thought he knew what he was talking about. But how could he, with all his knowledge, imagine that he could "take" my children and make them lose both their father and their mother in the same day? Was it possible that this well-intentioned specialist of the mind didn't understand that my children needed more than anything else my physical presence, my body? As I needed theirs. "To take" the children, to release me from my responsibility to them, isn't that the same as taking charge of all three of us, of reducing us to the stereotyped image of widow and orphans, weak and beholden to the authority that claimed us?

Later on, I learned that some relatives of my husband's patients named a small dead-end street in the suburbs "L'Impasse du Dr. Bertherat." Here at last was a gesture that seemed just, human. Defenseless before the bodiless mask of Authority, they had found this way of expressing that they too felt themselves on a dead-end street.

I reached out to just one person. Suze L. received me in her office, a small, quiet room that opens onto an unruly garden behind her house. She sat down next to me. She didn't touch me. She waited for me to be able to speak. Through a haze of images, of memories, I sought the clarity of commonplace words. I found: "I have to work. I have no resources."

"Yes, you do."

"If I could do your kind of work. Before leaving . . ."

"That's what you wanted to tell me?"

"You'd guessed?"

She didn't answer.

"Do you think I could?"

"I'll help you. You have to have a diploma. There are many things to learn."

"But what about what you can't learn? Serenity. Patience."

"You're mistaken. Serenity, as you call it, is something that I learned and it was the most difficult thing of all."

"I can't imagine you any other way."

"I was quick-tempered, even violent. Before."

"Before working?"

"Before being operated on."

She waited until I looked into her eyes.

"I was operated on twice. Breast cancer."

Not in that warm and solid body! It's not possible that death could have entered her body, too. Tears stream down my cheeks.

"It was ten years ago. I was still young. I took it all very badly. I felt damaged, morally too. I dreamed only of becoming once again the way I'd been before. I never imagined that I could become infinitely better."

I told her that I didn't understand. So she explained how, from her weakened and devalued body, she had built a fortress.

After her operation she couldn't cough or speak, she could

barely breathe without feeling pain. She suffered from sharp, constant pains in her shoulder, in her arm, on her entire left side. She couldn't move her arm behind her. "Why do you need to put your arm behind you? Isn't it enough just to be alive?" her doctor asked her.

But living under her body's oppression, she no longer participated in life. She felt isolated, humiliated, punished, alone with her pain. Like an animal in a trap, she saw no other way of escaping from her pain than by cutting herself off from the wounded part, leaving it behind her.

Then one day she read an article signed L. Ehrenfried. The body was described, not as a diabolical machine that holds us at its mercy, but as supple, malleable, perfectible.

She remembered that several years before, she had gone to see Mme. Ehrenfried, a specialist in problems of left-handedness, because she was afraid of misguiding her daughter, who couldn't make up her mind to be "a real lefty."

Mme. Ehrenfried had reassured her about her daughter. Then she'd suggested that Suze L. work with her. Thinking Mme. Ehrenfried meant that she wanted her as an assistant at the lectures that she gave to the parents of children under treatment, Suze L. declined and had never seen Mme. Ehrenfried since then.

But after reading the article she went back to that extraordinary woman who had fled Nazism in 1933 and found herself in Paris armed with a German medical doctor's diploma that was invalid in France. Alone, she came to understand that her primary refuge was her own body. Slowly she developed a method of what she called "gymnastics" for lack of a better word. Her reputation as a brilliant theoretician spread by word of mouth and soon she had hundreds of enthusiastic students.

Mme. Ehrenfried always worked one side of the body and then the other, for she'd discovered that when one side is fully alive, the other side cannot bear its inferiority. It becomes available to the teachings of the "better half."

Through Mme. Ehrenfried's method, Suze L. stopped being concerned solely with her mutilated side and started working on her normal side.

Contrary to classical gymnastics, which seeks to develop muscles that are already overdeveloped, Mme. Ehrenfried's gentle and precise movements helped her to loosen her muscles, to release an energy that she hadn't known she had. She learned that she had a shoulder, an arm, a whole side of her body that was strong and healthy, full of possibilities she'd never suspected. She learned to see herself honestly, without illusions, and to recognize at last the clumsiness that Mme. Ehrenfried had noticed years before when she'd suggested that Suze L. work with her. For she hadn't invited her to be an assistant, but a student.

Suze L., who'd never questioned herself about her body until it had become a source of pain, realized that until then her breathing had been superficial and irregular. She retained her breath just as she had always retained her emotions, her anger. Resigned for years to not knowing how to swim, she finally dared entrust her relaxed body to deep water and discovered that she did know how to swim and to find pleasure in it. She had been clumsy, unable to wash the dishes without breaking a glass or to raise a cup of coffee to her mouth without spilling it, but now her movements were becoming fluid and precise.

During the course of several months of intense work, she came to understand that her "good side" was better than she'd thought. But, most important, she discovered that her good shoulder was connected by nerves and muscles to the painful shoulder, that her ribs were connected to a spinal column whose vertebrae were articulated and mutually dependent. She understood at last that her energy, those waves of well-being that she felt animating the good side of the body, could and must pass over to the wounded side, which she couldn't leave for dead, which she had to make live as it had never lived before.

In the beginning her painful flesh resisted. It seemed to fear new suffering, to want to remain isolated, outside of the body's unity. She kept at it and soon her body, conscious of its progress, gained confidence. It even seemed to her that it was her body that took the lead over her will. Soon her body itself seemed to be trying to re-establish its unity, seemed to know better than she what it had to do.

"I began to go to all the work groups, five or six a day. It kept me completely occupied. My feet, my legs, my spinal column, my breathing, everything had to be worked on. It takes a long time to build a body that's aware of its strength."

"And now?"

"I still work every day. I try out all the movements that I have my students do. I must understand them with my body before I can make them understood by yours. Like all converts, my body wants to preach what it has discovered. But sometimes . . . Your new profession, you're going to discover, is not learned in books."

Her voice became softer still.

"It's work that makes exceptional demands on you."

I didn't understand. Not yet.

3

The
Music Room

At the age of thirty-six, I enrolled at a school to work toward a diploma. All the students lived in fear of the directress, a big, bony woman who had been an ambulance driver during the First World War. When I introduced myself, she tapped me vigorously on the shoulder and announced gruffly, "No sense going over what happened to you." She became a generous ally bent on my success.

I started to learn what lies under our outer wrapping: bones with their unbelievable number of tuberosities and tubercles; muscles—a skein of strings to unravel as you discover how they're attached and where they lead. The complicated nerve network. All of it shown in impeccable drawings done, not from a live model, but from a cadaver in the same Rouvière anatomy books that my husband had used during his first years in medical school.

The language was familiar to me, but at times I had difficulty understanding that those drawings, as rigid and technical as those of a machine, could correspond to the reality of the living body, which I now conceived as being in constant motion, charged with energy—a unified whole and not a collection of miscellaneous pieces.

One evening I suddenly interrupted my reading and called Mme. Ehrenfried.

"Come to my five o'clock class tomorrow. Come ten minutes early."

I hung up, struck by the musicality of her voice with its faint German accent.

The next day I discovered a solidly built, rather elderly woman with beautiful short white hair. Her penetrating gaze shot up toward the top of my head.

"I thought you were a blonde."

"What?"

"You have a blonde voice."

At one end of her large, bright room, with its view of the Montparnasse cemetery, there was a concert grand piano. The floor was covered with a great number of brightly colored rugs. And then there were the flowers, an abundance of flowers, on the piano and in tall vases in every corner of the room.

She turned around.

"Excuse me a moment. Sit down."

But there were no chairs. When she came back, I apologized for having arrived too early.

"Perhaps you'd like to prepare your lesson?"

"I never prepare my lessons! You have to work in relation to your students. You just need to look at them to see what they need. A lesson prepared in advance is a lesson bungled in advance."

"But how do you see?"

"First learn to see yourself, then learn to see others, and last help them to see themselves: that's a great part of the work you'll be doing."

"But what about the exercises?"

"The what?"

Her voice had risen an octave. I didn't dare repeat my question.

"That word doesn't exist in my vocabulary and shouldn't exist in yours either if you want to do good work."

Then, as if to make all the false notions I could have already acquired disappear once and for all, she looked straight at me and launched into an explanation of the basis of her method.

"Here we never mechanically repeat a movement. Forcing a body to act contrary to its unconscious reflexes accomplishes nothing, in any case nothing of lasting value. As soon as the attention strays, the body resumes its old habits. Academic explanations are forgotten immediately. What we do here is to *make perceptible to the student's senses* the defective posture and actions that he has been involuntarily executing for years. It's the sensory experience of the body that we're looking for. Have you noticed that there are no mirrors in my house?"

On her walls there are shelves full of very old leather-bound books, medical journals, music scores.

"The student must discover himself not from the outside but from the inside. He mustn't count on his eyes to verify what his body is doing. All his attention must be centered on the development of those perceptions which are not visual. In any case, the eyes can see only what's in front of them."

I nodded to show I was following her, but she didn't look at me.

"When the student finally succeeds in becoming aware of a clumsy movement or of the immobility of a part of his body, he experiences an unpleasant feeling. He's uncomfortable. His body wants to learn a better way of moving. It's up to us to give his body the opportunity to create new reflexes which will allow it to obtain the results it desires. For the body is constructed to function at its maximum. Otherwise it deteriorates. Not only the muscles, but also all the internal organs. But all this will become clearer later on. Just listen."

"I'll listen to you, madame."

"No sense listening to me unless you listen to your body as well."

The doorbell. Several people came in. In all, we were a dozen students. Later on I learned that some were orthodox physical therapists dissatisfied with the poor results they got with their patients. There was also a doctor who specialized in acupuncture, a teacher of mentally retarded children, and some crippled people who had come to retrain themselves.

Mme. Ehrenfried pulled a stool from the hallway and sat down.

"Stretch."

I didn't move. I didn't know what to do.

"Go ahead. Stretch in all directions. However you want. Like a newborn baby, like a cat."

It's not easy to stretch spontaneously. As a child, I'd been forbidden to stretch, especially at the dinner table. Mme. Ehrenfried came to my rescue.

"Lean forward a little. Raise your arms a little in front of you. Imagine that the upper part of your body is stretching toward the sky. Now bend your knees slightly. Your thighs, your legs are stretching toward the earth. Imagine that your waist is the borderline between sky and earth. What about your back? Do you feel it stretching?"

I nodded, but she wasn't waiting for an answer.

"Now lie down on your backs."

It seemed to me that standing up we'd already filled the room. The others more or less managed to create tiny territories for themselves on the rugs. I alone, backed up against the piano, remained standing.

"You're not as big as you think. Put your head under the piano. You'll have more than enough room."

That was the beginning of a lesson during which I discovered that my neck, which I'd always thought long and therefore elegant, was actually rigid and graceless.

Once I was lying flat on my back, Mme. Ehrenfried asked me if I could feel the weight of my head on the floor. I was about to answer that of course I could because I knew that the head is heavy; I'd even learned that the average weight of a human head is about eight to ten pounds. But I hesitated. I took the time to become aware of what I was feeling and discovered that I hardly felt the weight of my head on the floor at all. The entire weight of my head was supported by the back of my neck. Mme. Ehrenfeld told me to let my head become like an apple hanging from the tip of a branch. Sitting on her stool more than three yards from me, she helped me, through her words alone, to feel the apple become heavy, the branch become supple.

She gave me the feeling that my neck began not at the level of my shoulders but between my shoulder blades, and that it could bend forward "like the neck of a swan."

I liked the simple, old-fashioned images that drew all my attention to the part of the body in question. Later on, in my own groups, when I used certain versions of these movements to help my students to loosen their knotted bodies, I tried to use only words, to keep from touching them or demonstrating the movements to them. I wanted neither for them to imitate me nor for their bodies to submit to the pressure of my hands. I wanted them to be able to make for themselves the sensory discovery of their bodies. "If you have to touch, it's because you don't know how to describe," Mme. Ehrenfried used to say.

But words, too, are a delicate affair. If Mme. Ehrenfried had simply told me, "You have a rigid neck," I wouldn't have believed her because I thought my neck was fine in its usual position. If she'd told me that I was bracing myself against the blows that I expected or that I refused to grant my head its proper weight because until a few weeks before I'd counted on another head to think for me, I would have scorned her remarks. Or else I would have been frightened away by her perceptions, which I might have found all too valid. It's obvious to me that simple nature-related images are very helpful since they let you make your own way toward the realities of your mental and physical behavior.

During the course of that first lesson, I began to realize that the movements that Mme. Ehrenfried indicated to us were part of a coherent plan. Like musical notes which are added one after the other to form a scale, the movements of the head, the shoulders, the arms, the hips, the legs developed one after the other, revealing to the body the interdependence of its parts.

Another student, a young composer who had studied with her for several years, took the musical analogy even further. He said that her lessons reminded him of lessons in harmony. "Harmony," "harmonious"—those words had lost almost all their meaning for me because they'd been used to describe so many vague states. But for him the word "harmony" had kept its strict musical definition: the simultaneous combination of tones and chords. As my gestures became more "natural" because I was finally making use of the appropriate muscles and energy, I was able to understand that the movement of one part of the body is "lived" by the entire body and that the body's unity comes from the simultaneous combination of movements which don't contradict each other, but rather complement each other.

It was at Mme. Ehrenfried's that I learned to recognize and to respect the personal tempo of my body, to give it time to discover the new sensations it was looking for. "Using an arm or a leg in a new way requires the use of nerve commands that haven't been used before. If you rush, if you force yourself, if you sweat with exertion, you'll prevent yourself from hearing your body. The work we do here is delicate and precise."

For Mme. Ehrenfried, breathing is the basis of a harmonious body. We breathe in a stingy way, she said, "like the owner of a six-room apartment who lives only in his kitchen."

I considered myself more advanced than the others. Hadn't I already learned to teach breathing techniques to people with paralyzed abdominal and intercostal muscles?

Mme. Ehrenfried made us lie down on the floor.

"Don't do anything. Let yourselves breathe. That's all."

I inhaled energetically, swelling out my rib cage. Then I exhaled a little through my nose and immediately inhaled again.

"You won't die if you breathe like that," she said. "But you won't live either. Not fully, anyway."

I realized that I had the same problem as nearly everyone else. I didn't breathe out. I kept the air in my lungs, which therefore remained partially distended and were no longer in the habit of expelling air. For me breathing fully meant inhaling fully, swelling out by chest, making my nostrils quiver. But the most important thing is exhaling.

But how do you learn to breathe? Mme. Ehrenfried had no respect for any of the numerous techniques that make you immobilize your stomach or your diaphragm or teach you to "concentrate" and then let you fall into your old bad habits at the first distraction. Breathing should be natural. It's up to the body to discover, or rather to rediscover, its own personal respiratory rhythm.

But why have we lost our natural respiratory rhythm? Isn't it because from the first instant of our lives we hold our breath when we're scared or when we hurt ourselves? Later on we hold our breath in to try to keep ourselves from crying or screaming. Soon we find ourselves blowing out our breath only when we want to express relief.

Breathing superficially and irregularly becomes our most effective means of mastering our emotions, of suppressing our feelings. When our breathing doesn't supply us with sufficient oxygen, our organs function at a slower rate and our potential for sensory and emotional experience is reduced. And so we end up by "playing dead" as though our greatest problem were to survive until the danger—living!—was over. Sad paradox. Grim trap we don't try to free ourselves from because we aren't even aware of being prisoners.

How do you permit your body to rediscover the natural breathing rhythm it lost such a long time ago? Once again Mme.

Ehrenfried asked us to lie down on our backs and, this time, to close our eyes. Speaking very softly, rocking us with her words, she told us to imagine our eyes not as coming out of our heads, but as resting in their sockets, "like small stones that you'd let slip into a pond. Wait for the ripples to come to an end."

I relaxed and for a second I was far from my daily preoccupations. Just then I let out a deep sigh. And it is from that sigh onward, from that great involuntary outward breath, that my normal rhythm re-established itself!

Instead of inhaling copiously, exhaling greedily, and then inhaling again right away, my breathing came in three steps: (1) I inhaled, (2) I exhaled, completely this time, and (3) my body waited.

It waited to need air before inhaling again. I learned afterward that this pause corresponded to the time necessary for the body to use the supply of oxygen brought in by the preceding breath. For the first time in weeks, I felt a deep, inner peace. I started yawning, huge, uncontrollable yawns, as though I were finally quenching a thirst for air I had repressed for a long time, perhaps since my earliest childhood.

The most extraordinary thing is that once my body had rediscovered its natural respiratory rhythm, it kept it forever. The anxieties which had deformed my breathing before now gave way to the authority of my body, which had proved that it "knew what it was doing," that it was acting for my good.

From the moment that I brought my body a sufficient and regular supply of oxygen, from the moment that my lungs and my diaphragm could work at their maximum and, through their gentle and continuous movement, could "massage" my liver, my stomach, and my intestines, I noticed still other improvements. My appetite came back. My insomnia disappeared. I felt armed, ready to confront new responsibilities—although I didn't suspect yet how many I would have.

Much later, thinking about the work and the personality of

Mme. Ehrenfried, I could appreciate how her knowledge of the body-machine as it is shown in the Rouvière books hadn't prevented her from looking further, or, should I say, closer.

A doctor with an unusable diploma, she could "practice" only on her own body. She had understood that her health did not depend on the use of treatments that came from the outside, but on the proper use of the body itself.

4

The Haunted House

It's time to begin. Alone in the room where we'll be working together, I'm waiting for my first students. Four women. The day before I had seen each of them separately and briefly, just the time to look at them, to begin to see them. And to listen to them. The first three were very succinct. The fourth, V., spoke at great length, tirelessly.

A jerky delivery: a firework display of words that stop abruptly, just long enough for her to shoot a penetrating stare from behind her batting eyelashes, then take off again in a new stream of sparks. An unpredictable voice that slides out of range. Rather deep and pleasant, in mid-sentence and without any relation to its content, her voice rises, squeaks, chokes on itself, then comes down again as though nothing had happened.

She makes no effort to control her outbursts. She doesn't even seem to be conscious of them. She tells me that her psycho-analyst, who is one of my friends, recommended that she try my class. And since her analyst's word is gospel . . . I learn that she has an interesting job that doesn't interest her. That her marriage is falling apart. That she wanted a child but had never decided to have one.

"And I eat chocolate," she concludes. "Too much chocolate."

Struck by the ease with which she tells me about her uneasiness, I'm reminded of an actress giving a first reading, who hasn't gotten into her role yet. I don't know what my lines are supposed to be. But she's a soliloquist and doesn't expect any from me. She stands up abruptly, offers me her hand, then goes off leaving her voice, her voices, in my ear. But my eyes remember nothing, except that she had dark hair. Behind her screen of words, she had succeeded in hiding from me, in making herself invisible.

The meeting with H., the friend of a friend, was very short. To my question: "Why do you want to come to this class?" she answered with a faint accent I couldn't recognize: "To get rid of my belly." But she doesn't have any belly; she doesn't have any fat anywhere. A former model, her neck and legs are extraordinarily long. And extraordinarily stiff. But she doesn't seem any more aware of her stiffness than of the way she carries her head, which, when she leans forward, cranes out like a turtle's from its shell. Seemingly carefree, she flashed a professional smile at me and went out.

C., a longtime friend, tried her best during our first "official" conversation to talk about a serious accident she'd had in her childhood and an operation for a discal hernia several years before. She's still often in pain and doesn't like to talk about it.

N., a neighbor on my floor, wants to do "a little exercise" out of curiosity and because it's convenient. But halfway out the door she said she "forgot" to tell me that she often has pains in her back and that she goes to a chiropractor several times a year.

Since I had learned in school the importance of vertebral pathology, it seems obvious that I should give my attention above all to my friend C. and to my neighbor N.

Now here they are, all four of them in footless tights and solid-colored tops. Except for V., who's wearing a black sweater with white zigzag stripes. It hurts my eyes. But it's her eyes that are blinking. She moves forward cautiously in the empty room.

"I feel dizzy," she says.

Could there be too much light in the room?

Once they've stretched, I ask my four students to lie down on the floor. V. lets out an enormous sigh of relief. Lying down, does she find the (relative) security of the analyst's couch?

I ask them to imagine that they are leaving a bas-relief body-print on the floor, as they would leave a footprint in the sand. V. is no longer relieved. Her eyelids bat. She raises her shoulder, taps it, presses it against the floor. Suddenly, she sits up and grabs the toes of her left foot in both hands.

"I've got a cramp!" Then: "I get them all the time. At night. They wake me up. Why? Where do they come from?"

She seems astonished that I don't know. My other students are silent, concentrating on leaving their trace in the floor. My friend C. has taken off her glasses. It's touching to see her with her eyes closed, a fervent look on her face.

But V.'s miseries win out. Using her pathetically stiff toes as a starting point, my students sit up to work on the joints of their toes and feet. I force myself to impose a slow tempo, a gradual progression of movements. But I'm unable to ignore V.'s agitation, and the lesson goes much faster than I'd wanted it to.

I finish the lesson with a movement in which the back of the legs unbend like a cat stretching out to claw against a tree. Doing this seems to calm V. a bit. But once the session is over, we're all treated to a veritable explosion of words. We learn among other things that she is simultaneously the mistress and the slave of two cats (the claw image was significant for her). As my four students dress in the next room, I can hear V.'s voice over all the others, and even when they're in the hallway, waiting for the elevator.

Alone in my now silent room, I have a feeling of failure. I feel that I've been had. I'd meant to concentrate on those who were "really" suffering and all my attention had been grabbed by a young woman who hadn't even complained of any pain. And whose body I couldn't even remember clearly. In addition to her verbal armor, she used her intense stare to keep me from looking at her normally, and hid behind her irritating sweater. But when she was obliged to be silent, it was her body that cried out through its cramps, its batting eyelids. What unspoken long-buried truth does she think we want to tear out of her? What secret is she so avidly protecting?

Several hours later, I'm still preoccupied by the class, and by arm, shoulder, and thigh strain. My own! And yet I had only been conscious of using my voice. Motionless in front of my students, I hadn't even turned my back to them. Like a mother who won't let her very young children out of her sight for a second for fear that they'll hurt themselves or that some unpredictable danger will suddenly threaten them. And what if my work were dangerous? But I know perfectly well that the movements require no muscular strength, present no risk to the body. I would not understand until much later that vague first impression of being on dangerous ground.

I was getting ready for bed when the phone rang. A woman tells me she has a very painful stiff neck. I'm not sure who's talking. I think it must be N., my neighbor. But it's H.

She's at the door a few minutes later. It isn't pain I see on her face, but anger. In examining her, I notice that not only are her neck and shoulder muscles strained, but the muscles all along her back and legs as well. As I work on unknotting her severely contracted nape, she tells me not to spare her, to do whatever is necessary for her to be in shape the next day. She absolutely must be in shape. Why? Because she must get up early. She must do her shopping. She must prepare a meal. She must pick up her little daughter at the train station.

"She's been on vacation?"

"No, she lives with my mother. But the last Saturday of the month she must come to my house. She doesn't like to. She cries each time. But she must come."

"Ah."

"I must take her." Then she throws me: "Don't think I enjoy it." And she waits for my reaction.

I just keep working on the knots in her neck. She continues, "What I hate most is buying the food. I don't like cooking it either."

"Do you make her favorite dishes?

"Certainly not. She must learn to eat everything."

For a second, I imagine H. at the market doing her best to choose the least appetizing foods.

"Don't worry about overdoing it," she reassures me. "Tomorrow, you know, I must . . ."

I must. She must. Is it possible that this apparently independent young woman is so bound by duty that her body can't move any more?

"Do you often have a stiff neck?"

"No!" Then: "I don't know. I don't pay any attention. Yes, I do, I do have them. Every month. At least once a month."

I think I'm changing the subject by telling her that she has a nice accent, but that I can't identify it.

"Nobody can." A long silence. And then without my asking her any other questions, she tells me that she was born in Austria, but that she was brought up in Argentina. "In the Austrian way," she adds.

Even more than her father, it was her mother who taught her discipline. She learned to dive into freezing water, to walk for hours under a torrid sun, to sleep on the floor, to go across a vast tropical garden by night without a lantern, to minimize her injuries, never to cry.

"I wasn't afraid of anything, not even the hyenas that screamed in the night."

She doesn't criticize this education at all. But as she describes it with pride, under my hands I can feel the muscles I'd just loosened contract once again.

"Only snakes frightened me. They were all over the place."
Then: "My daughter's afraid of everything. Not even my mother
can do anything with her."

"How old is she?"

"Five years old already. It's a lost cause, I think."

She falls into a long silence and so do I. How can I explain
to this woman that the stiffness in her muscles is inseparable
from the stiffness of the education she's so proud of that she
wants to impose it on her daughter? She claims to be satisfied
with her upbringing, but her body protests. It pulls up short in
front of the obstacles she makes it her duty to overcome. She
thinks she loves herself. The only imperfection she sees in her
body is a belly that doesn't exist. How can I make her understand that she doesn't love herself and that she can love neither
herself nor her daughter until she becomes aware of the bound
and gagged body she now thinks she has to deny or defy?

Even if H. could understand and intellectually accept these
thoughts, they wouldn't help her. My work can only consist in
helping her to recognize the rigidity of her body. She consents
to come regularly.

Her stiff neck came back frequently during the first year, but
never as violently as the first time. In the course of months of
work with her, at times I thought I saw her mask of defiance
slip away for an instant, to be replaced by an expression of
introspection, of genuine emotion.

I never asked her any questions, but often when I looked at
her, I was reminded of this quotation from Wilhelm Reich:
"Every muscular rigidity contains the history and the meaning of
its origin. Its dissolution not only liberates energy . . . but also
brings back into memory the very infantile situation in which
the repression had taken place."*

* Wilhelm Reich, *The Function of the Orgasm* (New York: World
Publishing Co., 1971), p. 267.

And that danger that I'd sensed during my first class—might it not surge forth from our memories?

From my very first professional experience on, it has always been obvious that each new student has only partial, fragmentary awareness of his body. "One foot doesn't know where the other's going," you say to make fun of somebody. But the dissociation not only of the limbs but of all the parts of the body is very common and considered normal. We don't know how the parts of our body behave in relation to each other, nor do we know how they're organized or what their functions and real possibilities are.

At a very early age we acquire a minimal repertory of movements that we never think about any more. All our lives we repeat these few movements without questioning them, and without understanding that they represent only a very small sampling of our possibilities. It's as though we'd learned only the first few letters of the alphabet and were satisfied with the few words that we could compose with them. If that were so, not only would our vocabulary be reduced, but also our capacity to think, to reason, to create. When a human being uses only about a hundred of the words in his language, we say he's mentally deficient. The majority of us make use of a few variations of only about a hundred of the more than two thousand movements that the human being is capable of. But we'd never take seriously someone who suggested that we're physically deficient.

If we feel that we're not relating to our body, isn't it because we don't feel the relationship of the parts of our body to one another? As for the relationship between the head and the body, it's often inexistent, which explains why many people falsely believe in the separation of mental and physical powers. For many of us, the head is the head and the body is the body. And that's saying a lot. The body is often conceived as a trunk which has four limbs that are obviously connected to it, but we don't

really know how. We aren't fully aware that our head is connected to our spinal column, as are our arms and legs. For many
of us, the head and the limbs are, at most, satellites.

For these reasons we don't realize that we could increase our
intellectual possibilities by first becoming aware of how we turn
and move in space, of how we organize the movements of our
body. It doesn't even occur to us that if we were to improve the
speed and precision of the nerve commands between the brain
and the muscles, we would also improve the functioning of the
brain.

We don't make the connection either between our body
and our head considered as the "metaphorical" center of our
emotions and our memories. We freely admit that we need
time and maturity to "know where our heads are at"; we spend
our lives looking for the answer. But we ask our body, which
is no less mysterious, no less "ourself," which is inseparable
from our head, only the most superficial and misleading
questions.

The rigidity of our bodies and the restrictions imposed by
that rigidity cause us discomfort and sometimes severe pain.
Without help, however, it's practically impossible for us to
recognize and analyze the real causes of our distress. Its origin
is masked by a single detail that captures all our attention: a
stomach that sticks out, one shoulder that's higher than the
other, a painful toe—or else we're "nervous" or can't sleep or
have trouble digesting. Sometimes we can't see the forest for a
single tree.

That's why the deep desire of a person who comes "to do some
body work" rarely corresponds to the reason he expresses. Let's
look at some of the most frequent reasons: *to get rid of one's
stomach; to exercise because sedentary living isn't good for you;
to get into shape for vacation.*

To Get Rid of One's Stomach

If people pay so much attention to their stomachs, it's because they don't see much else. Literally. Human eyes are placed so that we have to look in front of us and at the front of the body. As soon as our stomach sticks out a little, we see it, and very often, whether it's fat or not, we see it as excessive.

Why? Let's go back to H., who wanted to get rid of a stomach that existed, I dare say, only in her head. We saw how her body rebelled against the training that her mother imposed and how, by her attitude toward her daughter, H. repudiated her own maternity. Doesn't belly mean "mother" to her? Doesn't she really want to get rid of her mother's influence and of her mother's presence within herself?

Let's not try to draw too many conclusions. But let's not keep ourselves from asking questions. Especially when we know that thousands of women dream of "flattening" their stomachs. They see their naturally round stomachs as fat. In the name of fashion, they're prepared to do anything to have just the kind of stomach which, by definition, they can't have: a boy's stomach.

As for men, they're often humiliated at having a "woman's stomach." Don't they want to be flat in the hope that when they lower their eyes, all they'll see is an erection?

It's possible that this flat image we want so badly corresponds not only to our hidden fears but also to the reality of the limits to our perceptions. Paul Schilder's very interesting experiments, which I've often had my own students do, show that we see ourselves in two dimensions and not three.

The experiment consists of asking a person to describe himself as though he were standing opposite himself and could see himself from the outside. He will describe an unmoving image, with no weight or volume, very like a reflection in a poorly lit mirror or like a slightly blurred, probably not very recent, photograph. By wishing ourselves flat, we might be trying to correspond to our superficial visual perception of ourselves. Wouldn't fuller perception lead us to a correspondingly fully alive body? In order to feel "full" of life and not empty, don't we have to have a sense of our physical volume?

Center of the body's gravity, the convergence point of its axes, the place where food is converted into energy, our first link, through the umbilical cord, with life, the stomach seems to be respected only by the Orientals.

In the West, our center has become a target—of our contempt. We think of the head as the capital of the body. Then come the heart, the lungs, the so-called "noble" section. And then there are the visceral organs, the belly, the genital organs and what is called in French the "shameful nerve" which serves them: the inferior section. Proud to have elevated thoughts and sentiments, we'd prefer to ignore our low-down sensations. We don't like to acknowledge the existence of our stomach when we see it or when it makes itself felt, usually through pain. I remember the advice of a teacher of "deportment" I had at boarding school: "If during the course of a dinner you suddenly have the runs or any other stomach pain, it's preferable to leave the table with your hand over your forehead to give the impression that you have a migraine."

Digestive problems, constipation, ulcers, one could go on forever enumerating the psychosomatic sicknesses situated in the "inferior section." We're aware of our stomach because we see it and because it makes us suffer. For seeing and suffering are the two principal means of perception for those who have only a partial awareness of their bodies.

All these considerations don't exclude the fact that veritably deformed and flabby stomachs, and the valid determination to reduce them and firm them up, do exist. But how do people go about it?

They pedal in the air; they do "leg scissors," "push-ups." In concentrating all their effort on their abdominal muscles, in seeing only those muscles, in having therefore only a fragmentary vision of their body, all they succeed in doing, more often than not, is damaging their lumbar region. Of course, by pedaling hundreds of times you can manage to have a hard stomach. But since your exercises force you to arch your back, which, in turn, pushes the stomach forward, you'll have a *big* hard stomach. But its hardness will last only if you don't stop "exercising," which is to say if you don't stop hurting your back. Why is this so?

Because you're only conscious of the effect—a flabby stomach —without looking further for its cause. Actually, it's not your stomach at all that deserves your attention. What's more urgent is to loosen the tension *in your back*. It's only after you've released the contractures of your back muscles that you'll see your stomach flatten. In the next chapter, there will be more lengthy explanations of the back, the part of yourself that's unknown to you, that escapes your gaze and therefore your control, that part that others see without you knowing what it reveals about you.

But start right now to understand the interdependence of the front and back muscles by doing this little experiment. Stand up with your feet parallel and carefully joined, the big toes touching each other, the inner sides of the heels, too. Make sure that the feet are in the axis of the middle of the body.

Let your head fall forward. The top of the skull should lead the movement, so that the back of the neck bends and the chin is close to the sternum. It's easy to describe, but you'll see that this elementary movement is not easy to do. Either your head just doesn't obey and doesn't fall forward at all, or else your neck can't come out from between your shoulders. Or if your neck does manage to bow like a swan's or a horse's, you feel pulling or even actual pain all along your back.

If you can make your neck bow forward, let the whole upper part of your back go. Your arms ought to hang forward like a puppet's. But now your feet want to spread apart. Why? To recover your body's equilibrium, it seems. But there's a more appropriate explanation that will be given later. For the moment, keep your feet together. And continue to come down. But don't strain yourself. Don't make any back-and-forth pumping movements to get yourself farther down. Simply let yourself come down as if your whole back were slowly being drawn forward by the weight of your head.

Look at how far down your hanging hands fall. Knee level? Calf level? Ankle level? All the way down to the ground? If your hands are touching the floor, look carefully at your knees; your eyes are well placed to do so. It's very likely that your knees are turned in toward one another. Are they completely "cross-eyed"? Look closely at your feet. The big toes diverge, accentuating an eventual hallux valgus, or bunion.

Are the palms of your hands flat on the floor, in line with the axis of the body? Are your knees joined, taut, and turned toward the outside? Are your legs straight, knees in a plumb line over the ankle bones? What about your head? Is it relaxed, hanging freely? Bravo! Now I'm sure that your stomach is flat, well-muscled, and solid and that the posterior musculature is supple and relaxed.

But maybe you abandoned this experiment immediately because you discovered straight off that you're "too short" by eight or twelve inches. Maybe you've already said to yourself, "I'm not supple. So what?"

So this: the stiffness you feel in your legs is that of the posterior musculature in its totality, from the back of the skull down to the bottom of the feet. It's not in front that you're "too short," but in back. The deviations of your knees and the joints of your feet are the proof. The bones adopt a slanted position when the muscles are shortened, and the joints are deformed when this shortening is transformed into a permanent stiffness. This shortening of the entire posterior musculature is the cause of that stuck-out belly you don't like.

Tension in the back of the thigh makes for a soft and cottony front of the thigh. Which you don't like either (without good quadriceps, you can't carry your head elegantly, either). The internal rotation of the knees is the cause of those fatty accumulations on your hips that massages can only temporarily dissolve. If you're flabby in front, it's because you're too tense in back.

These conclusions may surprise you, but I'll explain at greater length in the following chapter. I think, though, that you've already begun to understand that the classic exercises for building up your thigh and stomach muscles counteract the results you intended. You can see that you can't work separately on the one part of the body that seems to need it. On the contrary. The "defect" is only the effect of a cause that's located elsewhere and that is frequently hidden because it is, literally, behind you.

Perceiving yourself in a fragmentary way leaves you, therefore, as vulnerable as an ostrich and deprives you of the possibility of fulfilling all the resources of flexibility and beauty that reside in your body, which is, whether you know it or not, an indissoluble unity.

By palpating your muscles and taking time to understand what you feel, you begin to know your body better than when you relied only on your eyes. Perhaps this little explanation of the human body's organization and symmetry will help you better understand your own.

It was through a drawing made by my seven-year-old son of a man (or a tree) that I came to understand the analogy of our upper and lower limbs. We have one bone in the arm (the humerus, with a humeral head that joins the shoulder blade) and one bone in the thigh (the femur, with a femoral head that joins the iliac bone of the pelvis). The forearm and the leg have two bones each. The hand is made of twenty-seven bones and all their corresponding joints, which give it a very large range of marvelously precise movements. The foot is made of twenty-six bones and all their corresponding joints, which, normally, allow it nearly as many possibilities. (But how many of us have stiff, "clumsy" hands, and feet that seem to be cast in a one-piece mold?) Just like the branches and roots of a tree, the extremities of the human trunk ramify and become finer as they do so.

The cranial *vault*, the thoracic *cage*, the pelvic *girdle:* each is a "container," but they also have in common the fact of being connected to the spinal column.

What about the spinal column? It's a mystery for most people. They could know that they have thirty-three vertebrae because they remember having read or heard it. But when you ask someone to lie flat on his back and tell you how many vertebrae he feels against the floor, the answer usually varies from two to a dozen. We forget that the spinal column begins at the skull, that the first vertebra (Atlas) supports it. And that the back of the neck with its seven vertebrae is part of the spinal column. The dorsal region with its twelve vertebrae where the twelve pairs of ribs are joined is also often unknown, unless some vertebrae stick out and make themselves known in a painful way. The lumbar region seems to be the best known, certainly because people often have pain there. But it is generally in a circular arch and there's no question of feeling its five vertebrae while resting on the floor. The sacrum does rest on the floor. You can even sense yourself in painful and precarious equilibrium when you're lying on your sacrum. But the tiny coccyx isn't perceived at all unless you've taken a "fall on your tailbone." It is nonetheless very often ill-treated and is often in peculiar positions— "fishhook," "corkscrew"—which affect the rest of the spinal column.

It's very rare for people to recognize the similarities between their head and their pelvis, both of which are rounded and capable of rolling harmoniously toward each other, if no dead zone keeps them from doing so.

Sometimes those who have begun to work on their bodies become frightened (only they know why) and quit: "I admit

I've got a fragmentary perception of my body. Too bad for me. But it's not as if I had some kind of an illness."

I don't contradict them. I'm not there to be persuasive or to force them to learn. But sometimes I'm tempted to tell them that yes, partial perception of the body is like an illness—a mental illness.

What in a normal person we call fragmentation of bodily perceptions can become pathological. Not only are certain patients unaware of their body as a unity, as a precisely determined, unified place, but they perceive the parts of their body as physically separated from one another. A mentally ill person sitting at home in his armchair can cry out in pain because his foot was just "run over by a car at the Place de la Concorde." Or else he can request funeral rites for his arm, which just "died in its sleep."

Of course, a person who's not aware of his body as a totality or whose body has several dead zones isn't necessarily a potential schizophrenic. But he certainly has a high potential for physical illness since he neglects certain parts of his body because they don't exist for him, overuses others to compensate for the lack, and blocks the free circulation of energy necessary for his well-being.

But what is perhaps most serious is that his dawning illness, sneaky and often unsuspected, is contagious. Those close to him—his children, in particular—are the most vulnerable. How many deformities—stooped shoulders, crookedly carried heads, excessively arched backs, shuffling walks—that we prefer to believe hereditary, are really due to a child's imitation of his parents? When we refuse to become aware of our body, don't we abdicate a much greater responsibility than we have for ourselves alone?

But it's not just those who are aware of suffering from slight, everyday discomforts who give up working on their bodies. The most dramatic abdication I encountered was that of N., a fifty-year-old woman. She suffered from a very severe deformity of the spinal column which gave her a humpback, painful digestive problems, faulty blood circulation in her legs, swollen eyes, and splitting migraines that incapacitated her. N. brought a stop to our work together just at the moment it became obvious that she could be cured.

From the very beginning, she seemed to defy me to improve her condition. But at the same time she behaved as though she already had or had always had a normal body. She never looked straight at me. When she spoke she sounded bored. Her only subjects were her new clothes and her social outings. She had nothing to say about her body. It was not a subject; it was not the subject.

I treated her with the Mézières method, which I'll tell you about at greater length in the next chapter. For the moment let's just say that it's a natural method that demands the patient's awareness of his body and his total cooperation. But N. seemed absent from her body, to the point of never admitting she was in pain, even when I knew very well that what I was doing had to be extremely painful. Because of the gravity of her deformities and her own lack of participation, I was obliged to hire an assistant to try to somehow replace N.'s own presence.

After a year of weekly work, we were able to re-establish nearly normal blood circulation in her legs, restore some semblance of life to the dry, scaly skin on her back, clear up her digestive problems, and reduce the acuteness and frequency of her migraines. At each stage of her progress, N. became more aggressive. You would have thought she was angry at her body because it was cooperating in spite of her, because in the painful battle in which we were engaged each week, her body was on "my" side rather than on hers.

At the end of the second year of treatment, it became evident that the terribly exaggerated curvatures of her spine were changing. She had grown a little over half an inch. When she told me she'd had to have her clothes taken in, she said it with the same tone of reproach she used to explain that I made her "lose" two hours on the highway for each hour that she spent with me.

Then there was the session when she came to a decisive turning point. Her body yielded to our efforts; we even succeeded, if only for an instant, in holding it straight. Joyfully, I announced to her that we were on the verge of reaping the fruits of our labor, that from the next sessions onward the transformations would be visible and undeniable.

I believe this "encouragement" had the opposite effect from what was intended. In any case, the next day she phoned me to say she wouldn't be coming any more, she was too busy, and those two hours of driving . . .

For a long time I tried to understand. I told myself that the conflict was hers, that it was within herself and that I had nothing to do with it. But I felt concerned, frustrated, even at fault. As though I'd been an intruder in a house that was haunted by ghosts who jealously defended their powers. I asked myself a lot of questions about the role I played in that dark and ambiguous battle she had to lose in order to triumph. A battle in which she seemed to see me, not as an ally, but as an adversary that she could beat only through ruse.

"Be wary of the body," said a psychoanalyst who'd attended one of my classes a long time ago. "Our bodies belong to the realm of the mother. When you approach the individual through the body, you enter directly into the archaic layers of the personality."

Transference, countertransference—the stages in the relationship between patient and psychoanalyst are codified; that's the way it goes. But in work involving the body, in work that is essentially nonverbal, what words can you use? What code is appropriate, if not the secret, inexpressible code of feelings?

To Exercise Because Sedentary Living
Isn't Good for You

We've already seen how we have a partial perception of our body. We rely mainly on our eyes, our feelings of pain, and our sense of touch to inform us about ourselves. Because we've censored our sensations, because we've let our real dimensions diminish in our own eyes, we have the impression that we don't exist sufficiently. The more our bodies are strangers to us, the more we remain strangers to life. We lack confidence; there are so many things we don't dare do. We think we're incapable of doing them and very often we're right.

When we're dissatisfied with ourselves, what do we do? Instead of deepening our knowledge of our body and perceiving it from within, we add elements to its surface. Clothing, notably. We take great care to make a judicious, flattering choice of clothes which project a satisfying image of us, which distract attention from our physical defects or compensate for them. Instead of working on our body to develop its natural elegance, we rely on stylists to create ready-to-wear elegance. We put clothes on our back, but we don't carry them; they carry us. They hold us upright and they hold us together and give us an appearance of unity, a style.

With our knotted muscles, our skimpy movements, we feel cramped for room in our body. So we try to "spill over" beyond the limits of our body or to extend those limits so that our body will send back a more favorable image. We do this when we're alone, but above all we elaborate our image of ourselves when we're going to appear in public. Because our image of ourselves is also found and sometimes primarily found in the eyes of others. Thus, in order to be "presentable," we wear high heels, hairstyles that extend beyond the shape of the head, shiny jewelry, fake lashes, "falsies," and false smiles in synthetic colors. We redesign the shape of our mouth; we "put on" voices and accents; we try to walk like this or that movie star; we walk dogs chosen consciously or not to reinforce our image of ourselves, or children clothed and "trained" for the same purpose. By seeking innumerable ways to animate the exterior of our body, all we often succeed in doing is removing ourselves even further from its center.

"The image that expresses nothing is not beautiful," says Elie Faure. When the image of our body expresses only another image—one borrowed from the movies or from a fashion magazine—it can't have true beauty because it's removed from reality, from an authentic expression. It's this very expression which we do all we can to hide.

But it's precisely in this effort to hide ourselves, to protect ourselves, that we reveal all our vulnerability. For the image which we think we're projecting isn't necessarily the one that's being received by others. Between our intention and the effect that we actually produce there's often a gap. In our imperfect mask others may see only our need to wear a mask, our need to represent ourselves differently from the way we are. We think we're creating an illusion, but we're the ones who are living in the illusion of being seen as we want to be.

With all our accouterments, with all our so-called "second skins," we still feel uneasy in our first and only skin. Because we don't have the feeling of our body, we say we don't feel well. Not only do we not feel *well*, but many of us hardly feel at all! (This revealing double meaning exists in many languages.) We complain about having superficial relations with others. We find them secretive, inaccessible. But actually we perceive them no better than we perceive ourselves. If we can't "get to the bottom" of someone else, isn't it often because we float on the surface of our own reality? If we reproach someone with not knowing how or not wanting to put himself in our place, isn't it often because our "place" is poorly defined, our "living space" not lived in at all, and because we're in a false position with respect to ourselves?

Often we attribute our uneasiness to our sedentary way of life. Although the source of our rigidity and our lack of physical sensation goes back much further, we're not entirely wrong.

Immobility is, in fact, a major obstacle in the perception of the body. We carry around with us parts of our bodies that haven't moved in years. And the more dead zones we have, the less alive we feel.

It's only through activity that our sensory perceptions can develop. But not through just any activity. Not through mechanical activity, not through movements repeated dozens of times. That serves only to exercise our obstinacy, to dull our intelligence. Movement reveals us to ourselves only once we become aware of *how* we move (or don't move).

The case of B., one of the first men in my groups, illustrates several aspects of these problems. To my question, "Why do you want to attend my classes?" this man of about forty replied, "Because I feel ill at ease." That must have seemed too brief. He added, "From time to time, I suffer from lumbago."

Lying on the floor, he nervously drummed his fingers on his stomach. His uneasiness was visible all along his body, which had minimal contact with the floor. Because of the contracted muscles in the back of his legs, he had a hollow space behind his knees. His whole body, from the buttocks to the shoulders, was held up by his sacrum and his shoulder blades. I was especially struck by the position of his head: the chin pointed toward the ceiling, the back of the neck arched. I asked him to roll his head on the floor from right to left, from left to right, and to try to feel the weight of his head on the floor. No use. He could neither move it nor feel its weight. "It's empty," he said. He could move his head only by raising it. His jaw and neck muscles were so tense that all movement seemed painful.

I asked him to stretch out his arms and unbend his fingers. He immediately complained of "unbearable" pins and needles in his hands. I asked him to shrug his shoulders. He seemed to be making a big effort, but his shoulders hardly moved. "They're made out of wood," he said. He told me he'd been brought up in a family where the children were forbidden to shrug their shoulders.

We worked on his shoulders, slowly and at length. B. closed his eyes; he seemed absorbed in the effort of traveling backward through time. Toward the end of the session, I asked him to rotate his two shoulders. He smiled at last. The movement was feeble, but he could feel the difference. "My shoulders seem oiled now," he said.

That was just the first step in a very long process during which B., who had been aware only of a sort of general uneasiness and occasional lumbago, discovered through precise movements that his whole body was stiff and unfeeling. He even started to look for the reasons.

We had a private session in which we both noticed that he had difficulty spreading his arms out wide because of the retraction of his pectoral muscles. B. told me he'd always been ashamed of his narrow shoulders. He always wore padded jackets. He recalled that when he was a very young man he had been invited to a country house on a torrid summer day. He had sat by the side of the pool but had refused to remove his heavy tweed jacket. In love with his host's daughter, he didn't want her to see his shoulders.

Once he became conscious of his tensions, he no longer knew how to carry his head. It wasn't possible for him to keep his former stiffness, but he was still far from having found his natural ease. "I feel as though my behind is between two chairs," he said. As for the tingling in his hands, he thought this nervous manifestation came from the fact that although he wanted to hide himself, he was obliged to use his hands which, by moving in space, drew attention to him. When he could keep his hands motionless, he wasn't too conscious of them. But when he was called upon to extend them, they tingled in protest.

Body awareness is certainly a first step toward better-being, but it doesn't bring instant comfort. The work can be long and painful. "Pleasure and the joy of living are inconceivable without battle, without painful experience and without unpleasant conflicts with oneself," says Reich.° The work with B. is not finished yet but, as he says, "I make believe less and less."

In my work I don't try to be the interpreter of others' behavior or of their discoveries. And it's important that they not look for an interpreter in me. But sometimes my students do inform me that after having begun to live in their bodies, they feel ready to go into analysis. Others, who are already in analysis, have told me that they had reached a turning point or that their analysis, which had been at the same stage for months, was going into its last lap.

In any case, the simultaneous existence of mental and physical problems in each of us is undeniable. But it's up to the individual to feel that unity in his own way. I can only point out one of the paths: becoming aware of one's body.

Feeling uncomfortable and vulnerable in our skin, we lock ourselves in behind accouterments, but also behind the doors of our apartments. Not feeling "at home" in our body, we rely upon a more familiar interior. We all know people who are "sure of themselves" if they're installed behind their desks, who are the "life of the party" if they're giving it.

Often those who come to work on their bodies for the first time find dressing in unfamiliar clothing, being barefoot, lying on the floor, or finding themselves in an unfamiliar room a very trying experience. One of the most dramatic cases was a very courteous, elegant, middle-aged diplomat. Dressed in a pair of immaculate gym shorts, he lay down on the floor, was immediately seized with nausea, and had just enough time to run to the toilet. Afterward, he phoned me several times to tell me that he

° Wilhelm Reich, *La Fonction de l'Orgasme* (Paris: L'Arche, 1976), p. 160.

didn't have the courage to come back and hoped that I would excuse him. He also hoped, I think, that I would explain his behavior to him. But the explanation could only come from his own body, which he would have had to question through the very work he didn't dare undertake.

Our upbringing, the restrictions which from a very early age we impose upon ourselves to spare us pain and pleasure, are not the only obstacles to the development of our perceptions. Our contemporary environment and standard architecture also play their oppressive role. When we work all day and all year long under artificial lighting, we can't count on the sun's rotation to provide us with temporal reference points. Since neither light nor shade turn around us, our body is no longer modeled by a continuous play of natural light and dark. Our third dimension is flattened, our presence in space reduced. Artificial, unchanging light crushes us, erases us. It also deprives us of another proof of our existence: our shadow. When the natural tropism of our body toward the sun is atrophied, our "wholeness" and our "wholesomeness" suffer and a part of our instinctive life dies.

Crossing the vast entrance hall of a public building where no object is on a human scale makes us feel "lessened" and undermines our confidence. The individual has no place in an environment conceived for the purpose of speeding up the movement of the crowd. He is obliged to modify his rhythm in that space structured as a passageway, which leads only to a stairway or an elevator.

To assure maximum rentable space, in recent buildings the staircases are built in a column at the middle of the building. When we go up we have no outward view, no way of situating ourselves in space; we can't read our body compass. Literally, we don't know where north is. South either. If the stairway is circular and the stairs are all the same size and spaced at equal intervals, when we look straight ahead, we can't tell when we're coming to the last steps. Almost inevitably we hesitate, feel about with our feet, or we stumble before we arrive on the landing. And our uncertainty or our clumsiness negatively conditions our behavior once we've arrived at our destination.

As for elevators, they upset our spatial reference points, but, also, due to inner-ear irritation, our perception of our body's weight and the relationship between our head and our body. We have very complex impressions, which I will summarize briefly. As the elevator starts to go up, our legs seem heavier. At the moment the elevator stops, we have the feeling that our body is still going up and then comes down again. When the elevator stops, our body feels lightweight and as if it has grown taller. We feel as though the internal substance that gives the body its weight has detached itself from our feet, has risen to the upper part of the body, and wants to escape. When the elevator goes down, the body seems not only lighter but also longer, as though part of the head wasn't following the downward move-ment of the body and had stayed in place. The main point is that in the elevator our corporal unity is attacked and we suffer the unfavorable psychic consequences. *

We can recognize our alienating environment and even suspect that it was purposely conceived to intimidate us, but that's where we live. And in spite of everything, we want to live fully. But how? In the first place, shouldn't we become aware of our body as the first place of our life? Shouldn't we learn first to live within our body, to organize its movements from within and in this way to have at least the possibility of freeing our-selves from the intimidation of an environment organized for use by "society" but not by individuals? But in order to feel that first of all, and most important, we live in our body, mustn't we acknowledge, perceive, and develop our feelings?

* An elaborate description of these sensations can be found in *Image and Appearance of the Human Body,* by Paul Schilder (New York: Inter-national Universities Press, 1958).

To Get into Shape
for Vacation

Sports: a panacea. If we don't participate in any, we feel guilty and promise ourselves that we're going to start tomorrow, absolutely. While we're participating in a sport, we feel young, vigorous, in shape. Afterward, if our back and limbs ache, we say that we must have been out of shape to begin with, that we don't do enough. We don't look any further for the explanation of our discomfort—perhaps because we're afraid of finding it.

Since so many people feel compelled to meet the challenge of mastering a sport, it's more important than ever to challenge the value of sports. There is absolutely no sport that is beneficial to the whole body—except walking. No, I haven't forgotten swimming, which people persist in believing a "complete" and even therapeutic sport. As for the French national sport exalted by the Tour de France and fast becoming an international mania, it does have its charms and obvious ecological advantages —but bicycle riding is, in a word, frankly dangerous to your health!

But first let's talk about swimming.

Recently I was visited by an American friend, an eminent anthropology professor and a specialist in "kinesics," the new science of analyzing body language.

"Just look at that," he said, pulling on his spare tire. "I don't understand it. I swim an hour a day at the university pool. And I mean *swim*. Not just float. I time my laps."

"How do you feel?"

"Fine. I'm not sick."

"What about your shoulders, your neck, the soles of your feet?"

"Fine. I told you, I feel fine all over."

"No tension in your muscles?"

"Tension! Don't you see how my stomach sticks out! You can't tell me it's tense."

"I can make you acknowledge one tension that you're not aware of."

"But I just told you—"

"What about your jaw? If the muscles you use for chewing weren't in a state of tension, your jaw would hang wide open, wouldn't it? This is a 'natural' tension and I guess it's natural to be unaware of it. But over the years you've added a multitude of other tensions all over your body and you're unaware of those too. Look at how you hold your arms."

Just a few minutes earlier he had demonstrated his typically American walk with its free-swinging arm movement. But now that his body was no longer in motion, the stiffness in his shoulders and in his arms—held far away from his body—was just like that of any French draftee being reprimanded by an officer.

I told him just that. He protested. I asked him to bring his feet together and bend forward with his head lowered and his arms dangling. He was "too short" by about twenty inches.

"You see? It's my stomach that prevents me—"

"No, it's not."

He started to sweat. The front of his thighs trembled. As was to be expected, the muscles all along his back were hard as rocks. He stood up straight again, out of breath: "But I assure you, every day I swim for an hour against the clock."

"And against yourself. When you compete against yourself, it's your well-being that's the loser. Water can be a marvelous playground. It soothes, it relaxes, it carries us and makes us forget our weight, and sometimes our cares as well. You might say that it has the power to 'dissolve' our tensions. But if you transform it into a battleground, you'll always be the loser."

"That's just poetry," he said, annoyed.

"Then here's some anatomy. When you're in the water, you're

in the same position as the snake, which uses only its spinal muscles (those attached to its spinal column) to propel itself. Have you ever looked at professional swimmers? Under each arm, you can see a mass that, in extreme examples, looks like a bat's wing. This is the mass of the dorsal muscle. This muscle is frequently so contractured in professional swimmers that it pushes the tip of the shoulder blade outward, so that it juts out from the contour of the thorax when the arm is raised."

"Thanks for the anatomy lesson," he said. "But I don't see the point."

"The point is that all the movements in swimming—breast stroke, crawl, backstroke—call the back and spinal muscles into action. But if, a priori, if *before* you learn these strokes, your back and spinal muscles aren't long enough, elastic enough —and that's the case almost inevitably—swimming makes them contract and shorten even more. And that's true of all the other vertebral muscles. Swimming, therefore, makes you develop the muscles of the back of your body, precisely those muscles which don't need developing, which are, in all probability, already overdeveloped. And when the muscles of the back of your body are overdeveloped, the muscles of the front of your body can only be underdeveloped. And that, my friend, is neither poetry nor politics, but an anatomical truth of which I can give you numerous proofs if you're willing to start by working on your body."

"You mean that instead of solving my stomach problem by swimming, I'm making it worse?"

"Exactly."

I advised him not to force his body to master the classic strokes or to break speed records. The first thing was to work at loosening his posterior musculature, in order to give his body the possibility of finding a more equitable distribution of its strength. The next step was to entrust his body to the water, to pay attention to the sensations of his body in the water. Because it's through what the body already knows naturally—before having undergone any training—that the brain will learn. As far as speed and the beauty of the movement of the body in the water, they will come all by themselves, and there will be no need for a watch to tell you whether or not you should be satisfied with yourself.

Reich considered the bicycle a pitiful, masturbatory instrument. But there are more serious criticisms to make—and it's about time to make them. *The bicycle has none of the therapeutic qualities that are attributed to it.* To ride a bicycle without harming yourself, you have to have a body that's already exceptionally robust and well balanced. Why? Because you don't pedal with your legs, but with *your back.*

Just look at a cyclist in profile. With the nape of his neck hollow (he's obliged to raise his head to see where he's going) and his back rounded, he is putting to work the muscles of his lumbar region—muscles that are already very contractured because they are used constantly in our everyday movements. The stomach, however, is completely slack. (If you have any doubts, just try it and see for yourself. No use adjusting the height of the handlebars or the seat, which play no role in the basic mechanism of the movement.)

Thus, when you ride or race a bicycle, it's the posterior muscles, which are already excessively hard, that are put to work. And this causes their antagonists, the muscles of the front of your body, to become even softer. Result: on the one hand, a tightening of the muscles in the back of the neck and the lower back; on the other hand, a loss of tonicity in the abdominal muscles and a compression of the stomach which can lead to digestive problems (very common in professional cyclists). If you persist (because "the exercise is good for you"), you can also manage to cramp your wrists and your hands.

Practically without exception, athletes (and dancers) deform their bodies, sometimes monstrously, because they have only partial awareness of them. Since they don't understand the interdependence of their muscles and their antagonists, since they don't use the muscles that are best suited to the effort they want to make, they take their strength where they find it first. By forcing themselves, they have no choice; they're forced to hurt themselves. But forcing oneself, surpassing oneself, are often the rules of the game. Even when his goal is to beat his rival, an athlete out to win can rarely avoid "beating," which is to say "punishing," himself.

What, then, is the answer? "If even champions haven't found it, then maybe it doesn't exist," you might be tempted to say. The solution, the only solution, is not to put an end to sports, but to start at the real starting point: to start with the body and not with the sport. It's *before* you practice a sport that you must acquire muscular, sensory, and respiratory intelligence and use it every day and not only on vacation. Instead of limiting yourself to learned gestures, submitting yourself to the authority of specific training, you must give your body and your brain the possibility of inventing the most appropriate movements. Only then will you discover an aptitude for all sports, which you'll keep not only throughout your youth but for the rest of your life. No matter what activity is involved, your body will obey you, without trying to "revolt" afterward. "The more feeble the body is, the more it commands; the stronger it is, the more it obeys," said Jean-Jacques Rousseau.

Very recently, I saw a group of skiers getting off a train at a mountain resort. Their backs were humped, their necks sunk between their shoulders, their knees knocked against each other at each step or, if not, it was because their duck-walks kept their knees from knocking. I couldn't understand how people with such defective posture in "civvies" and on hard, flat ground, could possibly keep their balance once on the slopes.

Often they can't keep it at all. But sometimes they do. Not a real balance, but a precarious equilibrium with no harmony, no grace, and for which the entire organism pays the dues, for it's made of a multitude of muscular compensations. These skiers, who manage to go fast and mimic classical figures, are the very ones who will suffer afterward from exhaustion and painful stiffness. Which they'll consider normal. They'll even be proud of their pain, which they consider a receipt for so much energy spent.

And when their muscular contractions don't go away but, on the contrary, lead to "chronic" pains in their spine and in their joints, they'll be far from suspecting the origin of their distress. They'll say that they've fallen ill. But you don't fall ill; you slide. Sometimes very slowly, over a long period of abuse and lack of awareness.

"I've done nineteen sports," announced a fifty-year-old woman, as though she were challenging me. She seemed to have come to see me to make "anti-gymnastics" her twentieth discipline. "I have arthrosis in my neck," she said. "It's due to age."

I didn't contradict her, but asked her to lie down on her back. Her fanned-out ribs were painful to look at. Her thorax was rigid, as though she were incapable of exhaling the overload of air she'd accumulated over a lifetime of forced inhaling. Her feet were as stiff as a cadaver's; her chin, pointed in the air, seemed to be set permanently in an expression which revealed her desire to constantly surpass herself. I asked her to separate her fifth toe from the others. Nothing doing. I asked her to spread out all her toes. Not one moved, It looked as if she had on artificial toes.

Disturbed but wary, she asked me why it mattered whether she could move her toes or not (it's true that these tiny movements seem to have little importance). I explained to her that starting from this "paralysis" of her toes, especially the little and the big ones, which couldn't spread out from the axis of the foot, it was possible to detect stiffness and even a deformation of her entire leg. From the leg you could follow the problem up through the entire body, since everything is related. The back of the neck is responsible for the leg, the leg for the foot. By acting on the foot, you act on the neck.

She sat up and looked at her feet as though she were seeing them for the first time. I think that at that moment she began to understand things about a body she'd used less well than she'd thought. I took the liberty of telling her that she was wrong in attributing her arthrosis to age, that it is never time that rigidifies, but inappropriate use of the body. I recommended that we work together slowly and regularly so that she could learn to feel at ease in her body and no longer need to force it to obey her. She seemed quite disturbed and told me that she'd call me later.

I never saw her again. Over the course of the following months, she sent me several young athletes, but it seems that she didn't have the courage to question her own body, her own life. I think of her from time to time and I feel sorry for her. For it's never too late to offer your body the time to pause and re-evaluate itself. It requires a little bit of humility, but you're amply rewarded by the joy of moving with grace and precision, of making full, round gestures, of rediscovering all the sensations in a body free at last to live its real life.

"Every disturbance of the ability to fully experience one's own body damages self-confidence as well as the unity of the bodily feeling. At the same time, it creates the need for compensation," Wilhelm Reich so accurately observed.*

To compensate for their inability to fully experience their own body, to subdue the sometimes unconscious uneasiness that originates in their dead zones, some people resort to imitating. They perform stereotyped movements that are merely the more or less skillful imitation of some sports hero or other. This involves training the body, disciplining it, and not becoming

* Wilhelm Reich, *The Function of the Orgasm*, pp. 318–19.

aware of movements that one discovers and ripens within one-self by using one's brain as well as one's muscles.

But what is this satisfaction that people find in imitating "winners"? Isn't it a continuation of that of putting the body into ski equipment? With our sunglasses over our eyes, our poles in our hands, and our skis on our feet, our image of ourselves is enlarged and embellished, if not deepened.

Whether it be a tennis racket, a golf club, or a fencing foil, objects "lengthen" us and allow us to make longer gestures in space. (Adding a rigid object to an unsupple arm, however, lengthens only our rigidity.) When we imitate someone else's gestures, we become the other person in addition to ourselves. But afterward? Once we take off our skis and put aside our poles, we find ourselves alone—with our aches and pains. And with that feeling of sadness, of disappointment that the actor experiences in his dressing room once he's taken off his costume and his makeup after the last performance of the season.

Our need for disguise and imitation is so strong that we ask our children to satisfy it too. We claim we want to do only what's best for them, but often we act in their worst interest because we don't perceive their bodies any better than we do our own. We have difficulty recognizing a child's authentic body language—especially our own child's—because we have difficulty deciphering the messages of our own body. We censor our own gestures and body attitudes and refuse to see them in others, especially in our "doubles." We don't ask our children to be faithful to themselves but to an image that we choose for them and impose on them.

Since a stationary image would be the most convenient for us, we're forever telling our children to "be still." But for a child, to move is as basic a need as to eat or to sleep. His physical and also his intellectual development depend on it. For movement, before it becomes automatic, requires neuromuscular coordination and intense cerebral activity. A child's "agitation" is his way of investigating not only the external world but his own possibilities.*

When we scold a child for his physical activity, we reduce his field of experience, we impede the development of his intelligence, and we encourage him to repress the natural expression of his emotions. By giving the child, who has a natural gift for imitating, the example of skimpy or stiff movements, we teach him to deaden his feelings and we set him a trap of awkwardness and lack of confidence from which he'll have difficulty escaping once he's an adult.

Impatiently, we wait for our children to be able to express themselves verbally; we congratulate them for speaking like adults and being able at last to protect us from the raw truth that they had been continually trying to express through their body. We're reassured when, like us, they can use verbal language as a screen to hide their true desires, to modify their natural tendencies, to master their sensations. "Talk to me. Tell me what's on your mind. If you don't talk to me, how do you expect me to know what's wrong," say parents to children emitting corporal distress signals that they don't see.

Colette made these observations about children at the beach. The era has come to an end; the problem remains. "For every pretty child in the bloom of health, chubby-cheeked and bronze-skinned, poised confidently on two firm calves, how many little Parisians there are, victims of a mother's routine belief: 'The sea, it's so good for the children!' There they stand, half-naked, pitiful in their nervous leanness, with big knees, little cricket-thighs, stomachs sticking out . . . their delicate skin has darkened,

---

* Occasionally, however, the constant agitation of young children "who can't stay still" demonstrates neither an irrepressible curiosity nor an instability of character, but a severe contraction of the posterior musculature which the child is not conscious of but from which he is trying to free himself. Body behavior determined by the stiffness of the posterior musculature will be explored in depth in the following chapter.

in a month's time, to cigar-brown; that's all, and that suffices. Their parents think them robust, they are only dyed. They still have big rings under their eyes, their sorry-looking cheeks. The corrosive water is skinning their poor calves, troubling their sleep with a daily fever, and the slightest accident unleashes the laughter or the easy tears of those tiny nervous people dyed with chewing tobacco . . ."*

A Federal Body Expression Department hasn't been formed yet, but at times it seems that it can't be far off. Instead of doing sports or exercises, people rush to do "body expression," an ambiguous discipline somewhere between interpretive dance and psychodrama.

But if a priori we don't understand how to use our body, if our repertory of gestures and movements includes only a fraction of the possibilities of which the human being is capable, if until now we've used our bodies only to reduce, betray, or deny our sensations, then "body expression," like sports, can only be imitation, compensation, training. It's not surprising then that in corporal expression performances or classes, we see a kind of travesty, a stilted melodramatic representation of standardized ideas and, worse still, standardized emotions. Instead of imitating sports champions, we imitate actors or dancers or characters found in paintings or sculptures. It seems obvious that corporal expression, as practiced by adults who have only a superficial and routine knowledge of their body (and therefore of their life), can only be a bluff. For corporal expression to have any rhyme or reason, you must first become aware of your corporal repressions.

As for the new science which seeks to interpret body language or nonverbal communication, it seems very difficult to analyze

---

* Colette, *Les Vrilles de la Vigne* (Paris: Hachette, n.d.; "Le Livre de Poche" series), p. 221.

what a subject's gestures or body attitudes mean if you don't first know what he's physically capable of. A seated person whose knees, feet, and palms are turned inward can convey that he is refusing his interlocutor's advances. But his attitude might merely indicate that the extreme contraction of his posterior musculature keeps him from sitting any other way. Perhaps no matter what the situation is, this particular person always communicates the same thing: his inability to freely use a body that has been too stiff for too long. To study body language without taking into account verbal language is certainly valid but, before-hand, mustn't we learn the limits of our muscular vocabulary?

Before doing sports, *before* doing body expression, *before* interpreting the gestures of others, *before* declaring yourself "in the dark" about your children's behavior, *before* going into analysis, *before* resigning yourself to your sexual problems (we'll talk about them later)—body awareness is *preliminary* work.

As a painter prepares his canvas, a potter his clay, we must prepare our body before using it, before expecting "satisfactory results" from it. It is the state of the body a priori that determines the richness of lived experience. The awakened body takes initiatives, is no longer content to receive or to "put up with." When we live in our body, we give body to our life.

5

Françoise Mézières: A Revolution

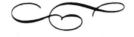

I almost never had the professional experiences that I just told you about. Toward the end of my studies I was ready to abandon everything, certain that I was on the wrong track. I'd wanted to do work like Suze L.'s and Mme. Ehrenfried's: help people to awaken their repressed, deadened body sensations, to rediscover their body unity and, through that unity, their health and well-being. But once enrolled in school, what I considered essential was never mentioned.

I found myself engaged in a program whose commendable goal was to teach us in three years the maximum of tested and approved techniques applicable to the therapist's work. We were constantly warned not to go beyond our limits. We learned anatomy, segment by segment, up to the neck. The head was considered beyond the limits of our work. Out of prudence, therefore, we were left in ignorance. *Primum non nocere.* We didn't risk doing much harm, but it seemed to me that we didn't stand much of a chance of curing either. Unless we came across a patient without a head.

As for my own head, I had the impression that it was no more than a card file where I classified information as (1) anatomical, (2) physiological, (3) pathological; in other words, the names, angles, and measurements of each deformity. By accepting this information, I also had to accept, for instance, that a splendid, smiling, and confident young woman could come into a re-education therapy room with a sore neck and go out totally demoralized, officially disabled, labeled with the name of a disorder, "cervicodynia," and holding a prescription for twenty thirty-minute sessions during which she would be forced to lift her head, attached to a sack containing a pound of sand, three hundred times.

In entering the re-education room, she had passed from the realm of the healthy to the realm of the sick. She had been reduced to a subject to be manipulated, or even less: a neck to be manipulated. Something within me refused this submission. But just where was this border between health and sickness and how could you avoid crossing it? How could you avoid letting yourself slip into the trap? I had no idea. I only knew that you mustn't let yourself be reduced to the name of a disease; you munst't let yourself be filed away in the pathological card file or you might never get out of it. Or if you did, it would be with the label "ex-cervicodyniac," which would be just a sword of Damocles.

But I didn't have time to take these thoughts much further. I was too busy taking exams, and completing my hospital training program, in which I learned the art of hitching pulleys at the right place when it was a matter of mechanotherapy, of preparing mud baths, of encouraging lumbago victims grimacing in pain to pedal on massage tables to strengthen their stomach muscles. On lucky days, I could catch a glimpse of a specialist in the hall and I was even able to follow him to the room of a "case" and, hidden behind his retinue, could retrieve a few bits of the wisdom that fell from his lips.

Then one day, because I'd been a very conscientious student, I was invited to a demonstration normally reserved for graduates. Profoundly distressed after this honor, I understood that I could accept neither the traditional concept of the therapist's work nor the concept of a sick person as a "nonperson," as a piece of body.

The subject of the demonstration was a machine, impressive in its dimensions and in the number of its levers, straps, and dials. We looked at it from all sides, then stepped back and waited in respectful silence. A nurse entered the room, firmly grasping a boy of seven or eight by the forearm. By way of introduction, she said: "A right dorsal, left lumbar scoliosis, x degree angulation." No family name, no first name, certainly no nickname—just the name of a deformity. Then the instructress took him by the shoulders and turned him around to give us a back view, a side view, a front view, while pointing out his deformities with a metal instrument she held in her fingertips. But I can hardly remember the boy's body. It was his eyes that impressed me, large brown eyes, wide open in terror. And justifiably so.

Once exhibited to the trainees, "right dorsal, left lumbar scoliosis" was taken in hand again by a nurse who slipped a jersey "tube" over his head, which was supposed to keep his hair back, and another over his thorax. Then they laid him down in the machine and attached him to it by his head, shoulders, waist, and legs.

The extent of the deviation of his spinal column had already been measured. Now they had to regulate the machine in accordance with those measurements. I couldn't help thinking of the machine described by Kafka in *The Penal Colony*, which was regulated to engrave on the body of the condemned man forced to lie on it the legal sentence: "Respect your superior." Could one force a little boy's body to obey this machine's admonition: "Stand up straight"?

The machine was put in operation. It pulled—a dry sound

like a slowed-down pendulum—on the boy's body. A flick of the lever and the machine came to a stop just long enough to check the figures. Then it was put back in operation. Stopped. Checked. Put back in operation. Stopped, checked, until the figures indicated that the work had been accomplished. Everybody's attention was on the machine. The child received only orders: don't move, don't cry or the machine won't be able to do its work. When, trembling and swallowing his sobs, he was taken off the machine, he was put immediately into a brace that was supposed to keep in place the rectifications the machine had just achieved.

When I left the room, I was trembling too and convinced of the uselessness and the cruelty of the methods I'd been trying so hard to learn. I knew that I'd just witnessed a particularly dramatic demonstration of those methods, but it was representative of just that contempt for the human being, of that confidence in mechanical treatments whose effectiveness could only be temporary. I felt impotent in the face of authority and could imagine no other alternative but refusing to be an accomplice, abandoning my studies. At that moment, a tall woman in a missionary nun's habit who had been at the demonstration spoke to me.

"Diabolical, isn't it? Fortunately that isn't all there is."

"What?"

"Fortunately there's the Mézières method."

"Never heard of it."

"Of course not. They're not about to teach it at school. Françoise Mézières's method is in absolute contradiction to everything we learn here. It's contrary to all their ideas on health and disease, all the techniques that they've decided once and for all to make official. Accepting Françoise Mézières means refusing the foundations of physical therapy as it's practiced today. To say 'yes' to Mézières is to say 'yes' to a revolution. So you can imagine . . ."

"But if her method is valid—"

"That's the worst part. No one, not one specialist has ever been able to refute her discovery and the method she derived from it. Those who have deigned to read her articles have tipped their hats to her with one hand and slammed the door in her face with the other. It's a grave situation. It's symptomatic not only of how medicine is run today, but of how in every sphere our lives are regulated by those in power. Today the only ones who can allow themselves to accept the Mézières method, the only ones for whom it's profitable, are the so-called incurables, sick people whose conditions have been worsened by inappropriate, repressive, inhumane treatment. Generally, the only practitioners who accept it are doctors who practice acupuncture or homeopathy, rebels who believe it's more important to respect the individual human body than the corporate medical body."

"What should I do?"

"Françoise Mézières has recently agreed to teach her method, but only to graduates. I advise you to finish your studies and then, if you want to know more about her method, you can go to see her."

I did just that. And now, for several reasons, I would like to describe her work—reserved until now for professionals only—in very simple terms.

It's obvious to everyone who has learned her method that it produces spectacular and lasting results, whether it's used to correct so-called normal ugliness or to cure major deformities. Yes, I said "cure": eliminate the cause of the deformity and not just temporarily attenuate the effects.

"We must not tolerate failure," says Françoise Mézières.

But the discovery she made twenty-five years ago and the method that springs from it and that she has never stopped exploring and perfecting are unknown not only to the public but to the great majority of therapists. Why? Because they can't be included in traditional study programs without overthrowing them, without obliging those programs and the vision of the human being upon which they're based to be seen in a new light. In order to see in a new light or to see at all, you have to open your eyes. You have to dare to observe the body in its totality, even if your observations contradict sacrosanct truths. And that is precisely what the "authorities," the specialists, are not yet ready to do. And so it seems to me that the only hope that a large public can benefit from Françoise Mézières's work lies in directly informing it about a discovery that everyone, including professionals, can verify with their own eyes, with the experience of their own body.

Let me introduce you, then, to a revolutionary technique, but also to an individual. Called a "genius" by her friends and a "mad genius" by her detractors, she is, like the method that bears her name, original, genuine, absolutely rigorous.

But let's start at the beginning. Armed with a diploma, I registered for Françoise Mézières's summer training program. After ten hours on the highway, the roads became narrower and narrower, the houses more and more scarce, the faces more and more inscrutable. Between the ocean and the marshes, an immense white sky over flat swampland and a road that narrows down to nothing: the end of the world, or its threshold?

At the edge of a pond, a large, low house in front of which someone is gardening. Hair as white as the sky. Pale eyes; a look that really looks. "Did you have trouble finding the house?" A deep, hoarse voice. If a tree could talk, it would have a voice like that.

She laughed at my tribulations, then stood up and offered me a smooth but very firm hand with joined fingers continuing the curve of the palm: a hand made for kneading clay, a potter's hand.

"You've come to the bear's cave." Actually I'd never in my life seen anyone move with as much suppleness as this little sixty-three-year-old woman.

On the other side of the house, other cars with license plates from several regions of France, and from Switzerland and Belgium. In all, there were ten specialists in physical therapy who would be participating in the month-long training program.

Here we are all together in a large room on the ground floor. It's absolutely empty. No machines. No special equipment. Not even a massage table. Nothing but a small rug. We're all surprised, maybe a bit suspicious, but what we're about to see and hear is going to disconcert us even more.

Françoise Mézières takes her place in the middle of the room and invites us to sit down on the floor around her.

"My friends, would you tell me what is the principal cause of the deformities that you're called upon to treat?"

At last here's something familiar, reassuring. Several voices call out at the same time: The force of gravity. Weakness of the posterior muscles. Rheumatism. Arthrosis. Arthritis. Asthenia. Decalcification . . .

Françoise Mézières fixes us with her pale eyes.

"My friends, twenty-five years ago, if someone had asked me the same question, I would have come up with the same asinine answers."

A heavy, stormy silence settles over the room. Françoise Mézières continues: "Classical teaching inhibits. It teaches us to measure with plumb lines and spirometers, to diagnose and then to treat, by using a rich panoply of clever machines, corsets, and braces, those deformities that are considered curable through therapeutic methods. As for disproportionate or awkward physiques, we must accept them as normal because they're 'classifiable' as recognized morphological types, or because ugliness is not on our official list of diseases. As for deformities called 'fixed' because of their extreme stiffness, even though they contine to get worse, we're told to entrust them to Lady Surgery or to their sad fate.

"I tell you that we must not arrest our gaze on every little twist and turn of the body. We must not close our eyes to reality in order to make it conform to our academic concepts. We must have eyes only for perfect morphology and we must let ourselves be guided uniquely by the elegance of forms."

The amazement in the air doesn't break the silence.

"I shall ask you to do something new. I shall ask you to observe. I shall ask you to touch with your hands and not with instruments. And then I shall ask you to believe not what you've read, but what you've perceived."

To train our faculties of observation, she asked us first of all to take into consideration the "sacrosanct truth" about gravity, which is supposed to pull us forward and against which we're supposed to resist by the intense action of our back muscles. All our troubles, therefore, are supposed to come from this strong action that our "weak" posterior muscles are obliged to exercise to support our spinal column and to keep us from falling forward. Consequently, strengthening these muscles to help them accomplish their principal task would be one of the most important functions of our work.

"In short, that's what you all learned, isn't it?"

Nodding heads. Then silence filled with distrust. "To start off, I'll ask you a little question. Why should this famous gravity pull us forward rather than backward?"

No one answers.

"Now I'm going to ask you to stand up and put yourselves in the position that you're used to calling 'vertical,' but which is simply biped. Fine. How do we maintain our balance? Try to observe yourselves. Maybe you'll realize once again what you must have discovered when you stood up by yourself for the first time."

By observing the movement of my own body I understood that I found and kept my balance by displacing my body's weight. I held my head and stomach forward and my lower back arched backward. I understood at last that the problem was not only to not fall backward, but to not fall forward either!

This displacement of the body's masses—head, stomach, back—accentuates our spinal curvatures, however. When the head is held forward, the muscles that are connected to the cervical vertebrae compress and hold the vertebrae in a concave arch—the way squeezing an accordion on one side makes the other side open its folds wide in a circular arch. The same thing is true for the muscles of the lower back in relation to the lumbar vertebrae. This curvature and the compression of the posterior musculature—the ransom paid for our equilibrium—can only get worse over the course of our lives.

The problem, therefore, is not at all the insufficiency of our posterior musculature, but its *excessive strength*. We mustn't, therefore, "strengthen" the back muscles, which are already excessively contractured, nor help them to better support the vertebrae. On the contrary. It's necessary to stretch the posterior muscles so that they'll release their hold on the vertebrae that are kept in a concave arch.*

Françoise Mézières explained that it wasn't just the effort to keep our balance that shortens our posterior muscles, but all movements of medium or broad amplitude executed by the arms and legs, which are interconnected with the spinal column. Every time we raise our arms higher than our shoulders, every time we open our legs more than 45 degrees, the back muscles become shorter. The shortening, the contraction of the posterior muscles, is always accompanied by an internal rotation of the limbs as well as a blocking of the diaphragm.

"It is against this shortening that we must fight, my friends. If, once you know that, you continue to want to 'strengthen' your patient's backs, to make them more tense, you are dangerous and irresponsible."

But the essential part of her discovery is that in eliminating the curvature in one segment of the spinal column, you displace

---

* The complete and exact description of Françoise Mézières's principles can be found in her own writings, intended for professionals. (See the Bibliography.)

it to another segment. When you correct the curvature of the lumbar vertebrae, you make the neck arch backward and vice versa. By making any one posterior muscle longer, you provoke the shortening of the ensemble of the posterior muscles, which behave as though they were a single muscle stretching from the skull to the bottom of the feet. This shows the uselessness of segmentary work that treats the body as though it were an industrial object composed of detached parts. It's absolutely necessary to regard the body as a totality and to treat it as such, while taking into account not a multitude of symptoms, but the *unique cause* of its deformities: *the shortening of the entire posterior musculature, which is the inevitable effect of the body's daily movements.*

She delivered this conclusion to us with an absolute certainty that came not from pride but from twenty-five years of professional experience. For since she had made this discovery, she'd never seen a deformity whose cause was other than an excessively contractured posterior musculature. For two years after making her discovery—which was contrary to everything she had herself learned and taught—she tried to prove to herself that her new observations were false. But they were true. All she could do was forge a work method which was not only based on the observation of facts, but was confirmed by a profound knowledge of anatomy, of articular mechanism and of neurology, an irrefutable, perfectly rigorous method, which seems to be extremely simple but which is extraordinarily subtle and adapts itself to the individual needs of each patient—a method that earned her exclusion from official strongholds.

As she spoke to us, I thought that it isn't just the individual who has a partial perception of his body but also gymnastic experts, therapists, doctors, and surgeons, who approach the human body segment by segment. And what if it were not just their professional training which inhibited their perceptions, but also their fragmentary approach to their own bodies?

As for this shortening which can only worsen over the years, wouldn't it have, parallel to the physical deformities that it caused, a disastrous effect on the individual's psyche? Isn't feeling cramped, physically reduced, the very opposite of a feeling of plenitude? Doesn't feeling crushed by your own musculature give you the feeling of being crushed by life? Doesn't liberating ourselves literally mean freeing our musculature so that we can reach the dimensions to which we aspire, our real dimensions? Isn't it better to be able to lengthen our image of ourselves through the "elasticity" of our muscles and our gestures rather than relying solely on the effects created by our clothes, our embellishments?

One of the trainees' voices interrupted my thoughts.

"You talk, Mademoiselle Mézières, as though the body were made only of muscles. What about deformities of the bones, the joints?"

Françoise Mézières explained to us that with the exception of fractures and some congenital deformities, it is the muscles that are responsible for the deformities of the bones and joints. When they're shortened, the posterior muscles pull on the bones to which they're attached and over a period of time cause the articular surfaces to be unable to work together with the exact precision that's necessary. The cartilage around the ends of the bones wears away.

Since it is the muscles that are responsible for the movement of the segments, Françoise Mézières advised us to be wary of X-rays that seemed to show permanently fixed joints which could only be treated, therefore, through surgery. For if the patient can move even very slightly, and if, in moving, he feels pain, then his joints, in spite of appearances, are not "welded" at all and can be treated by making the contractured peripheral muscles loosen their hold.

"The body is not made up only of muscles, but only the muscles determine the form of the body."

Then she told us the story of a very old woman who had lived in her village. She had Parkinson's disease with numerous complications and a severe scoliosis. Her body was bent in two, her head held always at the same angle. She slept bent, had not stood up straight for years. The day the old woman died, Françoise Mézières passed in front of her house. She went in and found the dead woman stretched out on her bed. Perfectly straight!

"Once she was dead, her muscles, of course, had released their hold on her bones and she could be stretched out without difficulty. In the cemetery, you know, all skeletons resemble each other."

Before talking at greater length about Françoise Mézières's rare faculty for seeing with a clarity unobscured by preconceived ideas, I would like to mention some of her other basic concepts, one of which is the search for the elegance of forms.

Perfect Morphology

Classical medical gymnastics is satisfied to analyze and classify the different types of morphology, which are considered constitutional and therefore irreversible. Whether you're ectomorphic, endomorphic, round, flat, or cubic, you are what you are. Our imperfect structure is considered normal because it's common. Isn't the beauty of just proportions, like health, an extremely rare gift of Nature? Beauty, because it is exceptional, would therefore be abnormal.

Françoise Mézières teaches that morphology shouldn't be the science of the classification of dysmorphisms, but the art of recognizing the perfect form, which is the only normal morphology. She taught us not to accept any treatment that is not directed toward that perfect form. For neither the importance of the

subject's deformation nor his age prevent him from being able
to approach that form in an appreciable way. To the stupefaction
of her trainees, she declared that neither morphological type,
even if it's hereditary, nor acquired deformities (with the exception of fractures and mutilations), are irreversible. She had
even concluded from experience that old people's bodies (her
oldest patient was eighty-five) are more malleable than young
people's and that she could obtain astonishing results with them.

Françoise Mézières's description of the normal body is that of
Greek sculpture of the classical period. Why not that of Hindu
sculpture or of French gothic art? Isn't beauty an idea as arbi-
trary and fleeting as fashion? Isn't the perfect form a question
of taste?

Françoise Mézières maintains that the only normal morphology is that which corresponds to the relation of the proportions of the body's parts to one another that characterizes
Greek art of the classical period. This art was unique in repre-
senting the human being as he *should be*—that is to say,
as he could be if he could give reality to his true potential. This
fulfilled human body is like that of a hero or a divinity. (The
great American dancer, Martha Graham, talks of "the divine
normal being.")

The Greek artist didn't attempt to express psychological,
mystical, or political contradictions—but rather a corporal and
moral unity that is not utopian but realizable and toward which
each mortal, out of self-respect, should direct himself. The
famous "serenity," which marks the works of the great Greek
period, is the expression of the achievement of this unity and of
the subject's perfect physical health, since, for the Greeks, there
could be no beauty without health. And there could be no
health without the beauty of just proportions.

The following descriptions will help you compare your body
with this normal image and understand that your real "defects"
perhaps are not those that claimed your attention until now.

Looked at from the front, the clavicles, the shoulders, the nipples, the spaces between the arms and the ribs should be symmetrical and on the same level.

Looked at from the back, the neck should be long and full (and not show two protruding vertical lines separating three grooves). The shoulder blades should be symmetrical and not stick out. The shoulders and hips should also be symmetrical.

When you bend your trunk forward, your head hanging loosely and your feet together, the spinal column should be totally and regularly convex. The knees should be directly over the heads of the anklebones (and not backed up over the heels). The knees should not be "cross-eyed."

It should be easy for you to stand up straight, feet joined together from the heel to the tip of the big toe. In this position, the upper inside part of the thighs, the inside of the knees, and the calves and the inner bones of the ankles (the malleoli) should touch.

The foot should broaden out from the heel to the ends of the toes, which should diverge and lie flat on the floor. The lateral edges of the feet should be rectilinear; the inside edge, notched by the arch, should be visible.

Any deviation from this description indicates a corporal deformity. And every deformity has its source in the excessive strength of the posterior musculature. When Françoise Mézières says "we're all beautiful and well-built," she means that we're all perfectible—once we're able to have a whole view of ourselves and once we're determined to model ourselves on that perfect morphology which is our potential reality.

But how many of us are attached to a detail we consider our "best feature" or our most charming characteristic, which, in reality, is simply a deformity that can only get worse over the years? A "seductive" walk that's merely the result of an elevated hip; stuck-out shoulder blades we find "charming" because they remind us of angel's wings; a gaze that's "interesting" only because the head is always cocked; a high, jutting behind which results from a dangerously arched lumbar region—our so-called charms are harbingers of future pain and distress. Only beauty can guarantee health.

Sometimes we acknowledge that a part of our body is ugly, but we don't take it seriously if we can hide it and if it isn't a source of persistent pain. The foot is an excellent example. Françoise Mézières talks about "those hideous pestles that Occidentals call feet." She adds: "You can't preserve the foot's perfect morphology when you wear shoes that constrain it instead of protecting it. Shoes should respect the contour of the foot and let the toes have the freedom of all their movements (modern aesthetics doesn't accept this, but can you imagine a Greek statue with pointed feet!). Since the arches act as springs, the inside of the sole of the shoe should be perfectly flat because the foot adapts itself to the ground and not the ground to the foot; the shoe conforms to the impression of the foot. Since the normal walk requires that the posterior-inferior edge of the heel hit the ground when the leg is in complete extension, there should never be a heel, no matter how small. However, no existing shoe style corresponds to these requirements."

But most often, when we are aware that a certain part of our body is ugly, all our effort is concentrated on the part that offends us. But our effort is fruitless. A good example is the great number of women who complain all their lives about the shape of their legs. They have thighs shaped like "jodhpurs"— heaviness of the upper thighs or a hollow between the insides of the thighs. No exercise or localized treatment gives satisfactory results. But they don't know why.

These deformities, in fact, are merely the result of the internal rotation of the knees, which in turn is the result of the stiffness of the whole posterior musculature. This stiffness is also the cause of the internal rotation of the shoulders, which roll forward and make the hands fall in front of the thighs when one is in a standing position. Actually, the middle finger should fall at the middle of the outside of the thigh.

Just as shoulders rolled forward influence the elbows and the hands, the internal rotation of the thighbone influences the knees and the feet and, depending on the case, can cause X-shaped legs, or legs shaped like parentheses, flat or hollowed feet, varus or valgus deformations, and all toe deformities. "To counteract ugliness, you must first counteract stiffness."

Still skeptical, one of the trainees thought he'd discovered a flaw in her theory.

"This is all extremely interesting, mademoiselle, but how do you account for subjects who are too supple? Hyper-elasticity does exist, after all."

Françoise Mézières smiled at him.

"Hyper-elasticity, my friend, exists only in dictionaries. In real life, there has never been anyone who was too supple." Before the trainee could protest, she added, "In a little while, I'll prove it to you."

Several hours later Françoise Mézières brought in a fifteen-year-old girl. Her doctor's diagnosis: hyper-elasticity with ligamentary weaknesses.

Smiling, the girl showed us her elbows, which pivoted disconcertingly. "That's my hit act at high school," she told us. Seen in profile when she was standing, her legs seemed to have slipped in their joints. Her knees were recurvate, which is to say that her kneecaps seemed to have backed up, pushing the knee backward.

Françoise Mézières asked the girl to bend forward. Apparently with the greatest ease, she placed her palms flat on the floor. She could almost do the same with her elbows. But the internal rotation of her knees was impressive: her kneecaps, instead of facing straight ahead, converged.

She lay down on her back and Françoise Mézières, with the help of two trainees, worked at stretching her posterior muscles.

A lot of work was needed to get the knees to turn back to the proper position. The adductors, muscles on the insides of the thighs going down to the knees, were shortened and hard as steel cables. "I hate putting on a bathing suit because of this hollow between my thighs," she tells us.

When at last we managed to lengthen the posterior muscles and, as a result, the knees could turn back into place, we discovered that it was impossible for her to extend her foot. The stiffness of the posterior muscles of her leg wouldn't permit it. We realized that we had encountered only stiffness and more stiffness. What had become of that excess suppleness she was supposed to have been suffering from?

Françoise Mézières taught us that if we knew how to take off our blinders, the relation of the forms of the body to each other would become evident. We would see the appearance of the anterior regions of the body change with the appearance of the back; that of the top of the body with that of the bottom, and vice versa. If the organism were treated as the unity that it is, it would be the end of casts, corsets, and arch supports, as well as of the panoply of weights, pulleys, and machines that are now found in therapists' offices.

While she was talking about the need, in our work, of using only our intelligence, our faculty of observation, our hands, and our own muscles, one trainee whispered to another, "You're never going to be able to get your money's worth out of all that material you bought."

Françoise Mézières heard. She interrupted her speech to say: "My friends, don't count on my method for making a fortune. In our work, we must count neither our time nor our trouble. We're not mechanics who work on an assembly line. Our work is long and difficult because even when only one part seems to require care, it's necessary to treat the body in its totality. It's work that demands all our attention and all our physical strength because muscles resist. They, too, prefer to keep their bad habits.

But we need moral strength as well. We're working against the current of erroneous but accepted doctrines and practices that resist all proofs of their inaccuracy."

She explained to us that the final goal of our work was to make the subject autonomous, master of his body. But he can win this independence only by becoming conscious of the organization of his movements. He must know himself and accept the responsibility of knowing himself better than anyone else can. Otherwise, he'll always seek authority elsewhere: in a doctor, in drugs, in a treatment. He might eventually revolt against the authorities that he himself has put in power. He might want to free himself from them, but he'll be unable to. His body will never belong to him if he doesn't take possession of it himself.

"Never seek to dominate another person's body, my friends. Our only pride should be to liberate it."

Respect for the human body, the determination to help an individual discover possibilities he didn't know he had, to make him more intelligent, more independent—after three years of official studies this was the first time these subjects were discussed. But who was this woman who spoke with such ardor regarding essential matters that no one breathed a word about elsewhere?

I'd learned that she was born in Hanoi and that she'd lived there until the age of nine. A bourgeois environment (her father was a lawyer attached to the French embassy), but with royal trappings. Twelve servants took charge of all the material tasks; at the age of nine she knew neither how to dress nor bathe herself. She was sickly, dyslexic. Her mother scolded her for doing everything backward "like a Chinese girl." Doing everythink backward, turning her back to what was acceptable and expected in her milieu, wasn't it that very faculty that allowed her to develop her method?

Later, when I studied acupuncture and the techniques related to it, I understood that if Françoise Mézières's method were to be placed in a context, it could only be Oriental. In looking at drawings of the "meridians," or the paths of energy in Chinese medicine, I was struck by the fact that all the meridians of strength (yang) were situated in the posterior portion of the body, from the skull to the bottom of the feet, and all the passive meridians (yin) on the anterior surface of the body. As in Françoise Mézières's work, in Chinese medicine, too, the yang should not predominate over the yin, and the body should be considered in its totality. This vision of a body whose health depends upon the balanced distribution of its energy is opposed to the Occidental vision of a compartmentalized body with a pigeonhole for every specialist and a specialist for every pigeonhole.

I remembered my first image of her, on her knees in her vegetable garden. The work that she'd just talked to us about required as much patience, as much humility as gardening. It would be as vain to try to accelerate the rhythm of the seasons, to hasten the ripening of fruit as to force a body to realize its potential. And like a seed, a body, if it has been well prepared, has its underground life. If during the weekly work session, the practitioner has been careful to orient a patient's body correctly, to prepare new ground where the body can develop and blossom, then the body will follow the positive impulse and naturally and independently develop in the right direction. Unless the individual gets frightened. Unless the responsibility of his independence and his maturity frightens him so much that he sabotages his own progress.

Later, when somebody asked her to sum up the essence of her work, Françoise Mézières found another image. She said, "I sculpt live bodies."

For twenty-five years she has used this anthropo-sculpture, whose only model is the normal form, to treat innumerable patients, including those declared "incurable" by specialists whose vision was limited to the segment of the body printed on their shingle.

During my training program, I attended a session that Françoise Mézières described in one of her texts: "Madame P., a physical therapist, arrives at a training program. We observe that her face is a little stiff and that there's something strange in her gaze. We demonstrate on her, as on each trainee, the principles of our method and conclude that she has difficulty drawing her left arm away from her body. Madame P. tells us that she was in an automobile accident two years ago. Her face had been cut and her visual field reduced. We palpate her neck: C2, C3, C7 are turned to the left. We work her neck very gently and the reaction (customary following the first sessions) comes immediately and very violently: chills, trembling, sleepiness. We lay her down, cover her, and she falls asleep. At the end of the afternoon, she tells us that she seems 'to see more widely.' We think it must be an illusion due to the perturbation since the experts, whom she had seen recently and for the last time, had declared that the deterioration of her visual field was absolutely irreversible.

"But after a second application of the treatment the following week, followed by the same reactions, Madame P. recovered her entire visual field . . ."*

What do these sometimes violent body reactions during or after a work session mean? Françoise Mézières explains that her method acts above all on the sympathetic and the parasympathetic systems—in other words, on the body's self-defense system. Forced to abandon its old habits, its reflexes, "the carcass gets scared." It literally trembles in fright; it tries to escape through sleep. Not being able to recognize ourselves any more, even when our familiar image pains us, is frightening. The unknown, whether it be death or a new life, repels us, makes us draw back.

---

* Françoise Mézières, "Importance de la Statique Cervicale," *Cahiers de la Méthode Naturelle*, No. 51 (1972), p. 11.

"What about respiratory exercises?" asked a young colleague who'd just finished her hospital training program.

"It is as absurd to learn to breathe as it is to learn to make your blood circulate," Françoise Mézières answered. "Breathing needs not to be taught but liberated. It's imperfect because it's blocked. And it's blocked by causes that are foreign to the respiratory function. It's blocked by the shortening of the posterior muscles. The only way to treat a breathing inadequacy is, therefore, to make these muscles supple."

She explained that even though the diaphragm may pass itself off as the victim of excessive curvature (lordosis), it is really the accomplice. For the diaphragm is one of the muscles which are inserted on the lumbar vertebrae and which contribute to retaining the lordosis. She told us to think of the diaphragm as the bottom surface of the thorax. As though it were the bottom of a box, its warping influences the walls and, inversely, the warping of the walls impedes correction of the adjacent surfaces.*

"All the movements that you use in classical therapy—forcing inhalation or pulling the spinal column back to 'open up' the thorax—only result in making the blockage of the diaphragm and lordosis worse. And you aggravate them even more when you make your patient raise his arms. All you have to do is look at the ugliness of the thorax during these exercises to understand that no improvement can come from them. No matter what the movement, if it makes the patient uglier, it can't be beneficial. We all have an innate sense of beauty, my friends. Never disavow it, and certainly not in the name of science."

---

* The diaphragm is a lordotic muscle by virtue of the insertions of its columns, set into the second and third (and often fourth) lumbar vertebrae, and by virtue of its psoatic arch, which extends from the transverse apophysis of the twelfth dorsal to that of the second lumbar. This is an unusual way to think of the diaphragm, since, from a classical point of view, only its respiratory function is to be considered.

Occult Pain

Françoise Mézières's teaching unraveled like a complex detective story. We were led to examine very closely the so-called evidence and to see that it hid instead of revealed the truth. In this way we observed that a flat foot, for instance, was not in itself "the guilty party," but that the foot was "the victim" of the internally rotated knee, which, in turn, was the victim of a muscular deformity of the back. To concentrate on putting the foot back "on the right path" would be to perpetuate the injustice of classical techniques and let go "scot free" a back which in the future would commit other "crimes" against the body.

But Françoise Mézières went much further. She refused to attribute to "Mother Nature" the physical inelegance, bizarre posture, cramped and stiff muscles which don't attract specialists' attention until they become major deformities. (For these slight deteriorations always get worse.) She helped us to look for the motives of these body reactions and to discover that they are, in fact, hidden. But instead of respecting their clandestinity, we were taught to reveal them and to treat them, even though they are invisible!

Thus we learned that there exist not only movements and physical attitudes that protect us from pain we're aware of, but also automatic defense mechanisms that protect us from occult pain. We know intuitively that if we use a certain part of our body, we'll feel pain even though we have no memory of ever having suffered pain there before.

To protect ourselves against this occult pain, we assume postures that create pains elsewhere. And it is these new pains that make us suffer consciously which we want to have treated. But if we want to get at the cause of the pain and not just the effect, we must look for and treat the occult pain.

An intellectual deduction too mysterious to be believable? To think that would be to misjudge Françoise Mézières, whose discoveries are always the result of meticulous observations and experiences in actual treatment.

Here is one of the numerous cases described by Françoise Mézières in which the "guilty party" was occult pain: "A young woman has been suffering from acute sciatica and lumbago for eleven years. No treatment (and she has tried many) has relieved her, and her case has been decreed incurable. For the last three months, she has been bedridden with an acute attack. We have to take her shoes off for her and carry her onto the rug.

"It is extremely painful for her to lie on her back and to have her legs raised at a right angle to the floor. The patient twists about and repeats: 'I'm in pain, I'm in pain.' We observe that her head constantly leans to the right. Entrusting her legs to the person who has accompanied her, we palpate her neck and discover that the third and seventh cervical vertebrae stick out on the right.

"As we work on the neck, we see the patient becoming calmer. Our helper is astonished to find that her legs, which had been pushing hard against her, feel lighter. Without trying to work on any other part of her body, we end the session and give our patient another appointment two weeks later. She's surprised at being able to stand up and put on her shoes herself. Seen again two weeks later, the patient was walking normally."[*]

Later on when I had my own patients and students, a dramatic incident reminded me of Françoise Mézières's work on occult pain and made me conclude that her discovery could also be applied to psychic pain.

One day, I had a young woman do some very small hip movements. Designed to reveal to her the potential suppleness of her pelvic region, these very gentle movements, which consisted of slowly opening and closing the legs, couldn't hurt anybody.

But suddenly she cried out in extreme pain. Moaning, she

[*] Mézières, "Importance de la Statique Cervicale," p. 8.

rolled over on the floor. I was all the more perplexed by what I considered a "hysterical" reaction because I'd always found her rather calm, attentive to the work on her body. The only thing that she'd complained about was a certain stiffness in her legs. She found herself "lubberly" in spite of her attractive appearance.

I covered her with a blanket and waited at her side. After a long moment, she got up without seeming to be in pain and apologized for her behavior, which she couldn't explain any better than I.

The next morning she called me on the phone. When she got home after the session, she had broken down. She cried uncontrollably. She trembled and felt she was suffocating. A crucial episode in her childhood, so painful that she'd totally repressed it, had loomed up in her memory. And all because of a slight hip movement!

As a child, she'd lived in a big house with a formal garden surrounded by a high iron gate with pointed bars. One day, she was playing with the caretaker's young son. To impress her or at her own instigation—she couldn't yet say—the boy started to climb up one of the iron bars. When he reached the top, he slipped. The point of a bar pierced the upper part of his thigh and the boy remained there, impaled, helpless, shrieking out his pain.

When the adults arrived, she was accused of having encouraged the boy to climb the pole. His pain therefore was her fault. The boy was taken to the hospital. When he came home, she was forbidden to play with him. She looked at him from afar, didn't dare go near him or even speak to him. After a while, the boy stopped existing for her. She forgot the incident or thought she'd forgotten it. She had led a normal life, had never suffered from anything except for that persistent stiffness in her legs.

By performing those little hip movements, she had for the first time moved the part of her body which had been a dead zone since the gate incident. The cry that she'd uttered was that of the wounded boy. The occult pain from which she suffered without suspecting it was another person's pain, but one for which she felt responsible.

She made rapid progress in the following sessions. Her hips and legs loosened up and at last she discovered the pleasure of swimming, running, dancing, making love—pleasures that she'd denied herself until then out of fear of awakening her occult pain.

During the course of the month that I spent with Françoise Mézières, all the accepted ideas that I'd just learned in school were overthrown. I mean exactly that. My ideas weren't simply modified or shaken or enlarged; they were overthrown, put out of use. I understood that it was impossible to reconcile Françoise Mézières's ideas with those I'd learned previously, impossible to adapt her discoveries to traditional practice. Her work constituted a veritable revolution, absolutely opposed to the *ancien régime*. Like the human body, her work is an indivisible whole.

But to fully appreciate Françoise Mézières, you must see her at work, body to body, with a patient. Throughout the entire session, she lives the body of the other person. She captures it in her gaze. She absorbs it through her concentration. She adopts its breathing rhythm. If a patient complains that she's hurting him, she replies, "I know; I'm suffering as much as you." She isn't talking simply about mental suffering but about the pain in her own muscles that never loosen their grip, in her own hands that won't be defeated by even the most resistant rigidity.

I find myself obliged to call Françoise Mézières's relationship with a patient "passional" because she seems to know exactly what he's feeling, because he grants her his absolute confidence even during long moments of extreme pain, and because her ambition for him—to be beautiful and free—is what we passionately want only for those we love.

6

Ancient Foundations

You exhaust yourself. Your energy, however, doesn't get exhausted. It keeps circulating. From the moment you're conceived until the moment you die. Your energy follows its natural course through the sealed labyrinth of your body until it reaches an obstacle. Then it falters, can't continue on its course, abandons it, and disperses itself. When this happens, you say that you're exhausted, that you have no more energy. But you do have energy. It's there. But you're preventing it from being able to be used in the most beneficial way. By obliging your energy to turn away from its natural course, you turn it against yourself.

It is our energy that gives our body its unity by animating our organs, each of which is itself always in motion. We've already seen how becoming aware of our body as a whole in which each element is dependent on the other is necessary to our own equilibrium and health. Now it's time to go further.

It's time to think about a reality that our way of life often makes us neglect. It's time to become aware of the relationship between the whole that is our body and the whole that is the universe, between the continual movement of our body's organs and the movement of the earth and the sun. In our era, we're so involved in making progress that we always look in front of us. We're so interested in specialization that our field of vision has narrowed. And what if we were to open our eyes to what doesn't "progress," what if we were to look around us at immutable phenomena?

We would observe that the cosmic rhythm that governs the cycles of the sun and the moon, day and night, the seasons, is the same rhythm that the movement of our vital energy obeys. We would observe that our body, without waiting for the approval of our "intelligence," recognizes cosmic laws and complies with them. When we've understood how our body lives its life, perhaps we'll be ready to help it function at its best by treating it and keeping it fit through methods that take into consideration the body's relation to nature.

Often those who live close to nature recognize more easily that their body is a part of it. My grandmother, for instance, who was often called upon by the women of her mountain village when they were ready to give birth, knew ahead of time which night she would be called: she just counted the phases of the moon. She also taught me that these phases disturbed the regularity of the ovarian cycles. She sowed her root vegetables when the moon was waxing and cut her hair when the moon was waning if she wanted the new growth to be abundant.

Orthodox physiologists have observed that each organ receives its ration of energy at a particular hour or season. The fact that asthma attacks occur most frequently at dawn is due not to chance but to the fact that the lungs are at the height of their activity at about 3:00 A.M.

Heart attacks are most frequent around noon: the hour of the heart's maximum energetic activity. The large intestine receives its strongest energy ration between 5:00 and 7:00 A.M., which accounts for the normalcy of morning bowel movements.

Recently, researchers discovered that energy—far from being

an abstract substance or a mystical concept—is a reality, which, though normally invisible to the naked eye, can be photographed. The work of Kirlian, the Russian scientist, gives visual proof of the existence of an energy force that animates every living animal or vegetable body. When photographed, this energy is seen as a brightly colored halo at the body's surface. It brings to mind the aureole traditionally painted around the heads of saints. Called an "aura," this halo loses its intensity and changes color when the organism is ailing. Other scientists have concluded that the parts of the human body that give off the brightest light correspond to the points that have always been used by acupuncturists.

But exactly what is being photographed? Where does this luminosity emanate from? From the organism's surface, from its skin. From its skin? you say. There is nothing more commonplace, more familiar than our skin. That's true. But our skin serves not only as an envelope for our internal organs; it gives them an uninterrupted surface on which the energy that animates them can circulate. You insist: Our skin is our skin and our internal organs are our internal organs; there's no confusion possible. I reply that the confusion arises precisely from this partial and separatist vision of the body. The unity of the body isn't limited to an awareness of the interdependence of the front and back of the body. You also have to understand the relation between the inside of the body and the outside. In fact, the internal organs "project" themselves on the skin and can be treated through the skin by techniques that have their source in the five-thousand-year-old traditions of Chinese medicine.

When the natural rhythm of the energy's circulation is disturbed by an internal cause—indigestion for example—or an external cause, which could be an abrupt change of climate, the healthy organism calls its own regulatory system into action. All you have to do is wait until you feel better. But sometimes this natural regulatory system gets overwhelmed; it becomes incapable of confronting the disorder. The energy flow detours and disperses. There is an overflow in certain areas, a scarcity in others. The energy fluid can no longer follow its natural itinerary. Like floodgates, "acupuncture points" are located all along this itinerary, and it is by the regulation of these floodgates that Chinese medicine insures the normal circulation of energy throughout the entire body.

But how can a tiny needle prick on a very precise point of the skin re-establish the interrupted circulation? Because the border that unites us with the cosmos—or separates us from it— is our envelope: our skin. It's at the skin's surface that the energy circulates and it's at the skin's surface that our organs—heart, lungs, loins, kidneys, liver—"project" themselves.*

Thus by using rigorous mathematical calculation to combine two or three points on the skin's surface (there are nearly seven hundred points in all), the acupuncturist can spectacularly relieve and heal ailing organs that are far from the needles planted in the skin. The art of truly great acupuncturists consists of working at a distance from the organ under treatment and avoiding direct local treatment. Contrary to popular opinion, the best results are not obtained with a large number of needles; artful acupuncture means combining the points in such a way that the fewest possible needles are used.

Acupuncture has always been preventive medicine *par excellence.* The mandarins of ancient China paid their doctors to keep them in good health and suspended their payments as soon as they became ill.

The use of needles should be reserved for acupuncture doctors. It is possible, though, to treat vertebral disorders and muscular contractures (and we've seen that according to Mézières everything can be a question of muscles) by massaging the points

---

* Energy, of course, also circulates at a greater depth, which explains why certain doctors use long needles that can pierce the body.

used in acupuncture. Called "micro-massage" in France and "acupressure" in America, this entails massaging with the thumb (according to the Chinese tradition) or the flat surface of the nail of the flexed index finger. Since among the points along the two sides of the spinal column are also situated the points that deal with the vital organs, the internal functioning of the organism improves when spinal disorders are treated. It's also possible in treating a hand or an arm to improve the functioning of the intestines or the heart or the lungs, whose meridians pass along the hand.

With the exception of some forbidden points that are never massaged, acupressure is not dangerous. It's important, however, never to use cream or oil, which act as insulators and nullify the effect of the massage. Don't ever massage an open wound, either.

In America, there are numerous acupressure manuals intended for nonprofessionals. It is true that acupressure produces spectacular results, but it's necessary to have perfect knowledge of anatomy and exercise extreme precision in locating the points to be able to get to the root of the ailment and to cure it. Nevertheless, here are some massages that can give you fast relief without medication. Naturally, it's always recommended that you consult your doctor beforehand.

Some of the points used in acupressure seem to be linked to the most diverse traditions with no apparent relationship to China. In France during the Middle Ages, for example, the undertaker, called *le croque-mort*—the "cadaver-cruncher"— actually did "crunch." In reality, he bit the tip of the little finger of the person who was presumed to be dead to be sure that he really was dead. It's well known that there is a reanimation point at the corner of the nail of the little finger on the meridian of the heart. In New York, the Iroquois are highly valued in skyscraper construction gangs because they never suffer from

Choe Keou. Reanimation point. Located at the base of the nose, above the upper lip. Pinch it hard between the thumb and index finger. Very useful in reviving someone who has fainted, this massage can be of great service while waiting for a doctor.

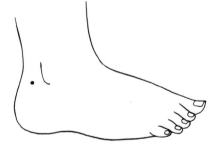

Kroun Loun. "Aspirin" point to relieve all pains. Situated on the outside of the foot, above the heel bone (calcaneum) between the outer anklebone (malleolus) and the Achilles' tendon. Massage it with your fingertip.

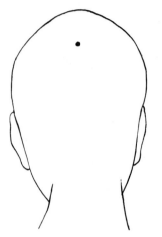

Paie Roe. Point for stimulating the memory and the intelligence. Located on the fontanel along the median line of the skull. Massage it with the tip of a finger. (It can hardly be called a coincidence that this point is also the "point of departure" for the tonsure of Catholic priests, the *chanka* of upper-caste Hindus, and the pigtails by which the Chinese were supposed to be pulled to heaven.)

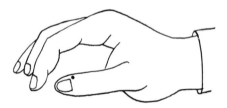

Chao Chang. Point for relieving sore throats. Located at the lower corner of the thumbnail (toward the index finger) of each hand. Press on it with the edge of the index fingernail. If you feel a strep throat coming on, swallow your saliva at the same time that you press on the point and repeat two or three times during the day. To be used also at the dentist's in moments of acute pain. (This massage is not, however, a substitute for a visit to the dentist.)

dizziness. It's been discovered that for generations Iroquois males were tattooed on the exact spot under the knee that corresponds in acupuncture to San Li: an important point in the treatment of fatigue, impotence, and also dizziness.

Through these brief descriptions of acupuncture and acupressure, you can see how it's possible to unblock energy and allow it to follow its natural circuit through the body's organs by acting not on the organs themselves but on their projections on the body's envelope.

There are other, perhaps even more astonishing, techniques based on the projection of the internal organs not on the entire surface of the skin, but on one part only.

It's told that Dr. Paul Nogier met a man he knew who was in great pain and bent over double with lumbago. In a gesture of comfort and commiseration, the doctor pinched his ear and was amazed to see the man, relieved and smiling, immediately stand up straight again.*

This doctor had just rediscovered an ancient treatment. The cauterizing of the external ear to relieve certain forms of neuralgia was practiced more than two thousand years ago. No one is absolutely sure if its origin is Chinese, Persian, or Egyptian.

After his empirical discovery twenty years ago, Dr. Nogier made a long series of observations, experiments, and verifications of neurophysiological data, and developed auriculotherapy. I shall not describe here the details of this technique, which should only be practiced by specialized doctors who use needles on points located on the outer ear. I would simply like to draw your attention to the resemblance between the shape of the ear and that of the fetus.

---

* For complete details, please refer to Dr. Nogier's book *Traité d'Auriculothérapie* (Moulin les Metz: Maisonneuve, 1973).

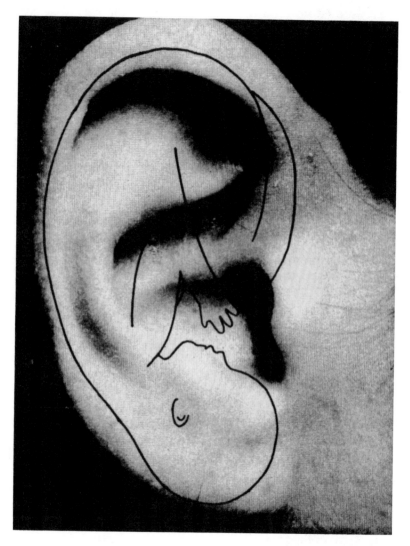

Photo: Martin Fraudreau

You can see that all the projections of the parts of the body are reversed: the lower part of the ear corresponds to the upper part of the body. The spinal column projects itself along the anti-helix; the projections of the feet, the hands, the limbs are just outside the antihelix; those of the vital organs are in the concha.

You might be even more surprised to learn that all the organs of the body are also projected on the skin of the soles of the feet, which we never even think about unless we have a painful corn or a callus (indicating that the body's weight is poorly distributed and that the foot is protesting against the overload).

Far from being "the object of constant care" (as it's defined in French army manuals), the foot is often the object of neglect and even scorn. But perhaps our contempt for the foot would become respect if we thought of the sole as a precise and complete miniature projection of our body in its entirety. Each foot is divided by a horizontal line that corresponds to the waist. The location of the projections of the organs on the sole of the foot corresponds to the location of the organs in the body. The heart, to the left in the body, is projected on the left foot; the liver, to the right in the body, is projected on the right foot. (You can find the same projections in your palms, but since your hands are constantly exposed, they are less sensitive.)

If you suffer from a serious or persistent illness, you should, of course, consult a doctor. But massaging the projections of body organs on the soles of the feet is a method whose source is as ancient as acupuncture and acupressure, and everyone can use it to relieve everyday pains. Thanks to *Stories the Feet Can Tell* by Eunice Ingham, this technique, called "reflexology," has had great popular success in America. Posters showing the soles of the feet, and the organs that are projected on them, suggest: "Massage a friend tonight."

Although it's possible to massage your own feet, it really is preferable to lie down, make yourself comfortable, undo tight clothing, and entrust your feet to a friendly hand.

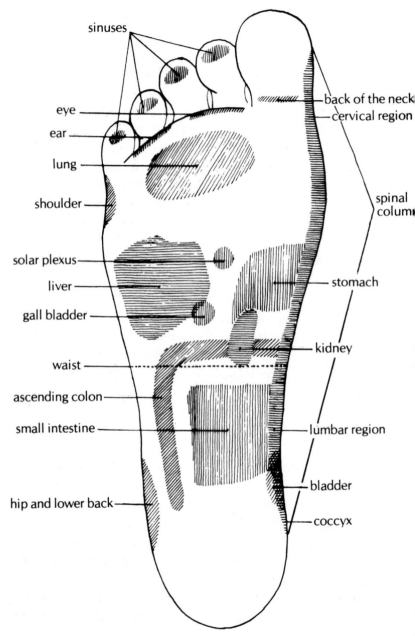

sinuses

eye

ear

lung

shoulder

solar plexus

liver

gall bladder

waist

ascending colon

small intestine

hip and lower back

back of the neck

cervical region

spinal column

stomach

kidney

lumbar region

bladder

coccyx

RIGHT FOOT

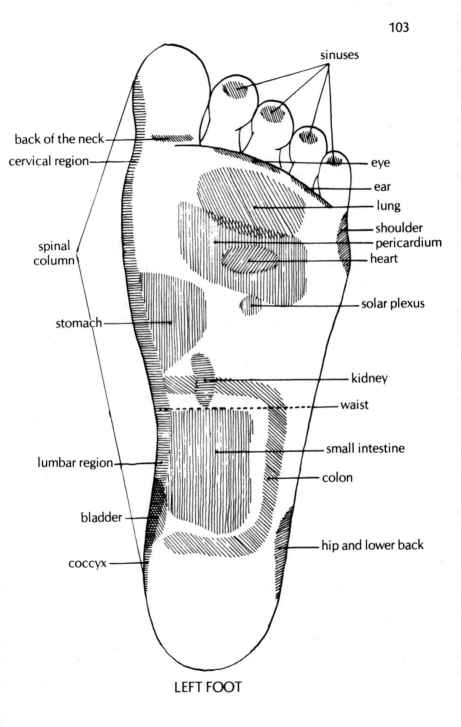

sinuses

back of the neck

cervical region

eye

ear

lung

shoulder

pericardium

heart

spinal column

solar plexus

stomach

kidney

waist

small intestine

lumbar region

colon

bladder

hip and lower back

coccyx

LEFT FOOT

To examine or to have someone else examine your whole body, all you need is a thumb. With the outer edge of the thumb (not the nail), rub firmly, horizontally, and without pressing too deeply the surface of the feet to find painful areas where it seems as though a crystalline deposit or grains of sand have formed under the skin.

This massage is not dangerous, but you should be wary of reactions. Too much zeal can result in diarrhea or a runny nose, for example. Nobody really knows why. But it seems entirely possible that stimulating too actively the circulation of the energy fluid can engender general excessive stimulation of all the organism's functions. The first exploratory massage, therefore, shouldn't last longer than five to ten minutes for both feet. Treatment massages shouldn't be repeated more than once a day.

Start with the big toe of the right foot. Continue toward the zones of the sinuses, the eyes, toward the ears, the bronchia, the lungs, the liver. Be careful with the liver. Located on the right of the body, a little bit above the waist, it's an important blood reservoir responsible for a dozen of the organism's vital functions. It's not uncommon to find its projection on the foot painful, even if the liver itself is not a source of pain. One of my patients, having massaged the liver zone for three days with a little too much enthusiasm, provoked such uncontrollable diarrhea on the fourth day that she couldn't leave her house. You must give the body time to adapt itself to change; never force it, even "for its own good."

You'll notice that the projection of the spinal column is found on both feet. I'm always amazed to find faithfully, along the inside edge, the correspondence of each contractured zone from the neck to the coccyx.

When you reach the zone corresponding to the intestines, be careful not to massage backward. Always massage clockwise in order not to disturb the peristaltic action of the digestive tube.

Thus, by applying your thumb against the sole of your foot

and by provoking the peculiar sensation of having a crystalline deposit under the skin, you can discover the deficient parts of your body, the aftereffects of illnesses, and chronic malfunctions. Not only can the present state of your organism be "read" in your foot but its future as well. For it's possible to detect a pain that indicates a predisposition to an illness. But diagnosis is for doctors. Be wary of amateur guesswork.

That's all for now. In these few pages, through the description of certain ancient therapies, I've tried to give you a new vision of the body. I hope that you'll try these methods and that, even if they seem improbable to you at the moment, their effectiveness will convince you of their profound value. For not only is it true the body is an indivisible unity inseparable from that of the cosmos, but awareness of this truth is indispensable to the body's equilibrium and health. I allow myself to express this certitude because my professional experience leaves me no doubt and therefore no other choice.

7

Keys, Locks, Armored Doors

A phone call from an old psychoanalyst friend. Before taking a young man into analysis, he wants to send him to me for some work on his body. What's this young man suffering from? Impotence, he answers.

Disconcerted, I reply that he seems to grant extraordinary powers to my methods. "We'll see," he says. "Keep me posted."

The next day, the young man came to see me: tanned, athletic-looking, about twenty years old, very pleasant. I would have thought him handsome, but something made me hesitate. Yes, he had consulted his family doctor; nothing abnormal as far as his body was concerned. So it must be in his head: so analysis. Faced with this obvious conclusion, he shrugs his shoulders. A small, skimpy movement. His shoulders seem shrunken, pulled forward by a knotted musculature. He holds his arms away from his body. I ask him to raise them. He has trouble raising his arms above his shoulders because they're restrained by his retracted pectoral muscles. The back of his neck is very stiff. He has difficulty turning his head from right to left. But there's something else. His gaze. It's as immobile as his neck. His eyes don't move independently of his head and his head moves very little. Is that why I hesitated to say he was handsome?

Not having any idea how to treat impotence, I decide to treat what I can and I enroll him in a group.

During the course of the following weeks, the extreme awkwardness of the upper part of his body becomes obvious when I ask him to move. Not only is he incapable of moving his eyes independently of his head, of turning, for example, his head to the right and his eyes to the left, but he can't even try to raise a shoulder without the neck and head moving, too—and in such a way that the shoulder movement is impeded! In other words, when I ask him to lie down on the floor and lift his shoulder as high as possible, making free use of all the parts of the body he needs to do so, instead of letting the head roll freely in the same direction as the shoulder, he turns it toward the shoulder and prevents it from·lifting. As for his pelvis, you would have thought it was welded. He couldn't lift it off the ground without his body, from the shoulder blades to the knees, rising with it like a stiff, hingeless board.

In group work he seemed very embarrassed every time we worked on the "inferior part" of the body. Sometimes he didn't move at all and just waited until we went on to something else. But he seemed to have no "complexes" about doing movements designed to make the "superior part" more supple. And so, for several months I helped him to unknot his shoulders and the back of his neck, and to recover the expression of his eyes. It was slow work, but little by little we both recognized his considerable progress. As for his impotence, we hadn't ever mentioned it since our first conversation. I'd completely forgotten that it was his original reason for having come, until the day my psychoanalyst friend called me back.

"Congratulations."

"What?"

"M. is cured. But he doesn't dare tell you yet."

"M.? The young man who had no expression in his eyes?"

"No, the young man who was impotent. Tell me what you did to him."

"I helped him understand that his head, his neck, his shoulders, and his arms were held in a tight harness that he alone could untie."

"I don't understand."

But I did. I'd come to understand at that very moment. The work done on this young man corresponded perfectly to a theory that I'd read but that I'd never consciously put into practice. Thus, like the "bourgeois gentilhomme," I had been using "prose without knowing it."

I said to my friend, "It's in Reich. In *The Function of the Orgasm* and in *Character Analysis*. No doubt you know them better than I."

"Wilhelm Reich? Oh sure. I read all that a long time ago. But you didn't go and lock up our friend M. in an orgone box!"

Still chuckling, he excused himself because his next patient had come, and hung up.

Wilhelm Reich. Dead in 1957 in a Pennsylvania prison to which he had been condemned for charlatanism, his theories on the circulation of energy (which he termed bio-vegetative currents or orgone) are now understood as corresponding to the circuits traced by traditional acupuncture points. Today the circulation of energy in every living body—animal or vegetable— is confirmed by incontestable neurophysiological proof. (See pp. 93–94.)

According to Reich, we keep our energy from circulating freely throughout our whole body by creating muscular "armor": stiff, dead zones, which encircle us, like rings, at different levels of the body. To protect ourselves against anguish as well as against pleasure, to protect ourselves against all feelings, we block the circulation of our energy, like M. for example, at the level of our eyes and our forehead, at our shoulder level, at the level of our stomach or our diaphragm (the case of the large majority of people who breathe superficially and deprive themselves of oxygen). And it is this blockage, this braking that is at the origin of our illnesses, our discomforts, our paralyses of all kinds.

But often we don't understand the relationship between our illness and our armor, which can be far away from the part of the body that's bothering us. As in the occult pain described by Françoise Mézières, we're conscious of suffering from one thing, but the origin of our suffering is elsewhere. As always, it's a question of finding and treating the cause and not the effect. Thus, M. complained of impotence, but his blockage (which he wasn't at all aware of at first and which his psychoanalyst, who was only interested in the "inside" of his head, hadn't noticed either) was located at and above shoulder level. Once the energy that had been blocked in the upper part of his body was freed and could circulate, the lower part of his body could put it to use, and his symptom, sexual impotence, disappeared. Reich says that it is "impossible to establish a vegetative motility in the pelvis before the dissolution of the inhibitions in the upper parts of the body has been accomplished."

M.'s case made me recognize that sexual problems aren't necessarily treated at the level of the genital organs or by unveiling the unconscious through the fragmentary means of words, memories, and symbols. The first step toward the solution of these very complex problems consists perhaps in just becoming aware of the body in its totality. For whether you call it orgone, vegetative current, or yin/yang, you must take into account that energy circulates for better or for worse in every living body and that when we block it, we suffer the consequences in one way or another.

After my "accidental" experience with M., I came to understand that I could apply Reich's work through the Mézières method. For the discoveries of Françoise Mézières—who knew little of Reich and wasn't particularly interested in his work—confirm certain of his theories and even take them further. Thanks to her perfect knowledge of the human body, Françoise Mézières could understand and prove anatomically that our physical distress and deformations come from a poor distribution of our energy and that our blockages, which manifest themselves in the front of the body, are caused by an excess of strength in our posterior musculature.

When Françoise Mézières tells us that we're ugly, ill at ease, and ailing because we hold ourselves arched backward, stomach pushed out in front, she describes the defensive position, which is for Reich exactly the opposite of the free and natural orgasmic position. (Isn't defending yourself exactly the opposite of letting yourself go?) The supple position of the earthworm or the rabbit, for instance, or of the embryo, which is a continuous forward curve, with the mouth and the anus coming toward each other, is possible only when all armor is abandoned (and when the posterior musculature is loosened). It is the only position, according to Reich, which allows the free circulation of energy and the undulatory movement of orgasm. Françoise Mézières described the equivalent of this position with her image of the healthy and supple body resting in a hammock.

Later on I had the opportunity to cure a case of impotence "without doing it on purpose" by using the Mézières method. A man of about fifty complained of pains in his stomach. He thought he was being "eaten away from the inside" by an unknown and certainly deadly disease because he had a "big hole" in the front of his body. He'd been sent to me for "remuscling of the abdomen." You could have put two thumbs between his large rectus muscles (muscles that are inserted on the sternum and the ribs and descend vertically to the pubis). His entire back was contractured and painful to pressure.

Actually, his "big hole" was even bigger than he thought. It began at the sternum and continued to the floor. For the posterior stiffness of his legs prevented him from bringing them together and they were always held apart. (But he hadn't noticed that!)

At the end of a year of treatment with the Mézières method, his dorsal and ischium muscles began to loosen their hold and his "mysterious illness" slowly disappeared. Little by little, the big hole became filled all along the front of his body. One day I congratulated him on his progress. He blushed to the ears and whispered, "But that's not all. After five years, I've 'rediscovered' my wife." He looked at me intensely to see if I'd understood. His words didn't surprise me, for his dorsal muscles had become more elastic and the adductor muscles in his legs had released their hold. The skin on his back had become smoother, more alive; the muscle tone of his stomach and the front of his thighs had improved. So why not his genital organs?

What about women? What about that avowed, unavowed, chronic, occasional, presumed, assumed, individual, universal problem, that "false problem" through which so many women express the deep truth about themselves: frigidity?

Women officially labeled "frigid" have been sent to me by doctors, gynecologists, or psychoanalysts. "Exercises won't do them any harm," they say. "They're distracting; they keep them busy; they make them use up energy." (Will they never understand that exercises are exactly what I do not do?)

Every day in my groups, in the street, at meetings, everywhere, I see women who certainly must be what people persist in calling frigid, although they don't openly complain about being so (at least not to me).

What's the matter with all these women? What is this famous frigidity? Frigidity, in a word, is rigidity.

No, my attitude is not supercilious. No, I don't lack compassion or understanding. No, I am not forcing myself to be simplistic. No, I am not disloyal. I am a feminist and I am for women's mobilization. But not only in militant groups. I am for the mobilization—the putting into motion—of each body of each woman. For it is only from within her own living, mobile body that a woman can find her strength, the possibility of her happiness.

Today a woman who proclaims "my body belongs to me" is often deluding herself. It's not because her body no longer belongs to him—the oppressive male—that her body necessarily belongs to her. To be able to say "my body belongs to me" implies that by becoming aware of her body a woman has taken possession of it. For her body to belong to her, she has to know its desires and possibilities and dare to live them. It is only once she lives in her body that a woman (or a man for that matter) refuses a relationship in which she is not "lived" by the other. Only when you know yourself profoundly do you refuse not to be "known" and do you seek at last to know the other.

Today when a woman believes that she's frigid she sometimes leaves the partner who is supposed to be the cause of her dissatisfaction and demands what she calls "sexual liberty." She looks either for more sensitive or more imaginative men or for other women and believes that through them she can discover her body, her real body.

Sometimes this change works. It really was the other person who was preventing her from becoming aware of herself. But that's exceptional. Most often, sooner or later she finds herself faced with the same problem. She's still not living her life because she's still not living her body. She hasn't chosen her new partners freely in terms of her real preferences. She doesn't know what she likes; the only thing that's certain is that she doesn't like her body. Dissatisfied and not knowing how to find satisfaction, she sometimes goes as far as to think that she's "out of her mind." But she'd be closer to the truth if she could understand that she's "out of her body."

What happens when a gynecologist sends me a woman who

says she's frigid even though he's found no physiological cause?

I enroll her in a group so that she won't feel isolated with her problem, and so that she can discover through movement how she lives or rather how she doesn't live in her body.

When she's lying on her back on the floor, one of the first things that I notice in a so-called frigid woman is that the movement of her ribs is almost invisible. She doesn't breathe. The diaphragm is stiff, knotted in back and immobile in front. You'd think that she has practically never put it to use. She doesn't offer herself the oxygen necessary to produce a sufficient amount of energy. Her tiny, minimal energy circulates so poorly throughout her body that she often says that she has no energy or in any case not the normal dose. As though energy came from the outside and she wasn't receiving enough. But you produce energy. As for oxygen, the combustible element necessary to the production of energy, it's not received at all. It's taken. You take it. Like you take pleasure.

I remember Mme. Ehrenfried's answer to a girl who complained of frigidity and asked if there weren't something she could do. Mme. Ehrenfried raised an ironic eyebrow and, on a long exhalation, told her, "Breeeeeathe . . ."

According to Reich: "Deep expiration brings about spontaneously the attitude of (sexual) surrender."[*] Anybody can prove this to himself. Exhale slowly, fully, and your pelvic region will start to roll forward—if you're willing to admit that you have a pelvic region and that it's mobile.

But let's go back to the group and to our frigid woman lying on her back. I ask everyone in the group to bend their knees and place their feet flat on the ground. Then to roll the pelvis forward toward the ceiling. The frigid woman is in total confusion. Like M., the young man with no expression in his eyes, she gathers her strength, pushes against her feet, and lifts up her

[*] Wilhelm Reich, *The Function of the Orgasm*, p. 298.

entire body, from the shoulder blades on down. If she's very ambitious, she lifts her body from the shoulders on down, from the back of her skull. And the pelvis? Suspended, rigid, it's somewhere in the middle of that long board she calls her body.

We start again. I ask everyone to lie flat on their backs again, knees still bent, feet still on the ground. I ask them to take their time, to find their pelvis—by using their hands, if they have to. Where does it begin? Where does it end? Where is it attached by muscles and bones to the rest of the body? How do its joints work? I wait. I see that they're fidgeting, moving around, that some look perplexed, that they're making a great effort to concentrate. I ask them to roll the pelvis forward, just the pelvis.

The frigid woman doesn't move. Her pelvis can't move forward independently of her thighs or her abdomen. Not only does it not move forward; it moves back! Her back is arched, her retracted pelvis refuses to move forward and upward. The natural orgasmic position, which is a continuous forward curve, an undulatory movement which brings the head and the pubis toward each other, is beyond her possibilities. She can't do it; she doesn't know that she can do it; she refuses it. Her pelvis doesn't seek to be full. On the contrary. It's not surprising then that she says she feels "empty." It's not surprising that she doesn't feel fulfilled, not to say overflowing, with life.

Moving the pelvis from right to left, from left to right, that she does know how to do. She does it when she walks and sometimes in a very exaggerated way, "like in the movies." She knows that wagging her behind is supposed to be feminine, sensual, and that by arching her back she attracts stares. She's willing to receive attention. Receiving is what she's looking for, what she wants out of life. But being just a receptacle is not a way of life—in any case, it's not a way for a woman to lead her real life. And when she realizes that she's not living the real life of a woman, she says she's frigid. But I say that she's rigid, retracted, refusing, rejecting, and, in a certain sense, reactionary.

I say that being able to articulate the empty word "frigid" won't get her anywhere if she doesn't know that her pelvis is articulated. And if she doesn't know that her pelvis, which shelters her *potent* genital organs, can come forward and *take* pleasure.

Take pleasure. An appropriate expression at last. Pleasure is taken. Like power, the real kind. Not the kind that's extorted from someone else and that deprives him of his own. Not the power that's bestowed on you if you're willing to receive it. To take pleasure, to take power, that is to say, to assume and exercise your own power over life and over your life, you must first of all take cognizance of your body.

But isn't it incongruous to talk about the power of the female body? About its potency? Doesn't potency belong only to men, since when a man is deprived of it he's called "impotent"? We never call a woman "impotent." When the energy charge, the spontaneous movement, the vital force, the orgasmic power of a woman are inhibited, we say she's "frigid." As though a woman without these impediments were only "hot," rather than potent. Why do we have a temperature criterion for women and not an activity criterion? And why do today's women, who reject so many "phallocratic" terms, still agree to call themselves "frigid"? How can they be made to understand that the woman's power that they demand, that they wait for the masculine world to grant them, can be found potentially in the body of every woman—and that it's up to the woman herself to discover this power and dare to exercise it?

But let's go back to the group and the effort to help the rigid woman, the impotent woman, to become aware of her body, of her sexuality.

We work on trying to liberate the pelvis. It's long, very long work and sometimes we don't get anywhere. But when the rigid woman begins to find, to feel joints that she hadn't known were there, when she begins to be able to move even a little bit, she suddenly finds herself in distress. Her dry throat, her moist palms, her cold sweat reveal the panic she feels. Finally freed of her old defenses, she feels vulnerable, she no longer recognizes herself, doesn't know what body she's living in. Sometimes her fear and her spontaneous (and momentary) rejection of her new condition are expressed verbally: "I didn't come here to learn belly dancing . . ." Or: "I saw a stripteaser once, the most vulgar . . ."

(These reactions remind me of the story about the early career of Elvis Presley, called at the time "Elvis the Pelvis." He was the first person, the first white person at least, to sing while behind his guitar his freely—some said frenetically—moving pelvic region rocked and rolled. An American student told me that Elvis Presley's first appearance on American television during the fifties caused an uproar. The cameraman, who had at first photographed young Elvis full-length and then in a close-up on the middle of his body—with the intention of showing his hands on the guitar—immediately aimed the camera at his face, where it stayed for the whole number. The next day, polemics in all the papers. For and against "lasciviousness" during prime time; for and against the "censorship" imposed by the cameraman!)

Sometimes the woman who had been rigid doesn't try to defend herself at all. She doesn't become indignant, doesn't censure herself. She very simply permits herself to discover her body. In the middle of the group, she remains alone, amazed, happy, in the special silence of those who are at last attentive to what their body has to tell them.

But it's not solely in the genital organs that sexuality is discovered or "treated" because it's not solely in the genital organs that it's situated. The body is a vast sexual network. To believe that sexuality is limited to the sex organs is to have a fragmentary vision of the body that is particularly dangerous.

Recently in my groups, we've been working on the head and its orifices. I will ask my students, for example, to close their mouths and to breathe only through the nose. They do it. Nicely, politely, methodically, and soon they've had enough. They get bored. They start to look at me as if to say: "So? What next?" I ask them if they feel something. No, they don't feel anything; there's nothing to feel. What about the air? What? The air. In your nostrils. The air that's going through your nostrils. Oh, yes. Where do you feel it? At the tip of the nose? Toward the eyes? They make faces; they sniff; they start to play with two thin streams of air as if they were playing a musical instrument. They play as they must have when they were tiny children. Some of them close a nostril or put a finger in it. They discover that they have two holes in their noses and that air goes in and that they can feel that it enters and that they can feel that it comes out. It's nothing at all, but for some people it's a revelation— and it's upsetting. They cross their legs, blush, try to hide their embarrassment, behave like the adolescents they once were. They've discovered that there are two holes in the nose and that air goes in and comes out and there they are sitting differently and looking around furtively and not knowing what's happened to them.

I take advantage of the situation. I ask them to relax their jaws, to leave their mouths open. Some resist from the first: "We'll drool." I tell them that drooling isn't so terrible. I ask them to stick out their tongues. I see tiny pointed tongue tips sticking out from between pinched lips. I tell them that a tongue is long, that they should let it hang out to its full length. No, much longer than that. Fine. And now, point the tongue toward the chin, under the chin. And now toward the nose. And now toward the right cheek, the left cheek. And now have the tongue complete the nose-cheek-chin-cheek circuit in a continuous movement.

Very few people consent to try immediately. Instead, they use their tongues to complain: "I'm getting all wet." "It hurts." "We really look bright, don't we?" Most of them, however, do end up by making the effort. More or less. But there are always a few people who categorically refuse. Their jaws locked, an expression of anger or distress on their face, immobile, rigid, resolutely armored to the teeth, they wait for the session to end. And sometimes they never come back.

The body knows that it is a whole, that one opening evokes another opening, that a sensation in a head orifice provokes sensations in the genital orifices, that becoming aware of one salient part—nose, foot, hand, tongue, phallus—leads to awareness of another. But if you don't want to admit what the body is saying, then you can take your time, you can take all the time of your life to try to gag it or to deafen yourself to its messages.

Let's go on. I ask my students to lie on their backs and relax their jaws again. In the meantime, some have understood that the jaw resembles the pelvis in its possibilities of movement and that it too can be held in retraction, locked into a position of recoil, of fear. This association may or may not facilitate the release I ask for. But let's say for now that they do manage to relax. Then I explain to them that this time it's a matter of feeling the tongue in the mouth, of feeling the width of the tongue, the thickness of the tongue at rest in the mouth.

At first, they don't know what to do with their tongue. They flatten it against the roof of their mouth or they draw it back toward the tonsils. But little by little, they let it live its real life of a tongue at rest, which has nothing else to do but swell, spread out, and fill the mouth until it has no more room and overflows.

When this happens, often a deep, thick silence fills the room. Eyes close. Bodies grow heavy and flatten out against the floor. Even the body of the impotent woman, if ever she has allowed herself to become aware of her tongue in her mouth. (If we do the rolling motion with the pelvis at this time, there is frequently less resistence.) Once I had a pregnant woman do the experiment of the tongue becoming thick and wide in the mouth. Later on, she told me, without explaining any further, "It helped me give birth."

Work on becoming aware of body orifices doesn't end, however, with the head. Recently, in a group attended that day only by women—one of whom was "officially" impotent and had been in analysis for several years—I proposed that we work on the "inferior" body orifices. I decided to take their silence for consent, and said, "Open your three orifices."

Seeing that they were unanimously perplexed—didn't they know they had three?—I added, "The anus, the vagina, the urethra. Open all three together. Wide. Wider. Now close them. Tight. Open them again, but slowly, widely. Feel that you're controlling your muscles, that you're making them make regular, precise movements." I assured them we weren't concerned with accomplishing superhuman feats (like the yogi who is supposed to be able to "drink" with the urethra), but with making them aware of their normal muscular power, with doing consciously the movements that they did, or didn't do, automatically.

Naturally I couldn't verify their efforts with my eyes, no more than my students could with their own. (Doesn't the faulty knowledge that women have of their own bodies also come from the fact that they don't see the intimate parts of their bodies unless they decide to look at them, that they don't touch them directly with their hands unless they decide to do so? And that from their earliest childhood these visual and tactile explorations are discouraged?)

I've had many proofs of the effectiveness of these movements (which one student called "sexercises"), but I must admit that some students—even longtime, faithful ones—don't understand a thing. One example was a very lively girl always dressed in the latest style whom I overheard complaining to a friend after a group session: "I really like coming here. But it's not erotic. She never talks about our breasts."

As if eroticism could be localized! As if the center of eroticism could be anything but the body in its entirety! I know that just about everything was "retro" that season, but had she adopted the mammary fixations of the American films of the fifties to such a point? Of course, the breasts "count." They have top billing on all lists of erogenous zones. But to become aware of the erotic potential of the breast, you don't have to take a course. A cool wind that blows by, a hand (even your own) that touches them lightly (even accidentally) suffices.

At the next session, I couldn't resist the temptation to give a little speech. I explained that here we became aware of the body through muscular movement and that we weren't directly concerned with the breast, because a breast is skin, fat, and glands. By wanting to "fortify" the breast or keep it from sagging, by doing standard contracting and stretching exercises, all you can do is develop the pectoral muscles—in other words, inflate the muscles behind and above the breasts. Result: a muscular chest and breasts as flaccid as they were to begin with.

Instead of fixing your attention on the breasts themselves, the important thing is to be able to see them in their "environment," particularly to consider them in relation to the shoulders. By unknotting the trapezius muscles, by letting the shoulders broaden out, you modify the position of the breasts, lift them, and improve the harmony of the proportions of the upper part of the body. As for the firmness of the mammary gland, no direct work on the breast itself can influence it. For a breast to be firm, for it to be well irrigated by good blood circulation, the entire organism must be healthy.

The extreme seriousness of the problem of sexual impotence—like that of fragmentary awareness of the body—became clear to me in treating a person suffering from very severe deformations: Mlle. O.

Her face was round, smooth; the expression of her eyes naive, innocent. I didn't have any idea how old she could be when, at our first meeting, she asked me to guess. Taking into account some white hairs in her long chestnut curls, her rather flabby body, and her prim, old-fashioned clothes, I guessed she was about forty. Her eyes lowered, her lashes batting, blushing with pleasure, she told me that she was fifty-nine. I found it sad rather than flattering to have a face of a young girl at fifty-nine, but I didn't say anything to her. She gave me a note from her doctor and, while I was trying to read it, started to relate the story of her life in a monotonous voice, as though she'd already told it many times before in similar situations. She lived with Mama, who was still in good health thank God, because somebody had to do the shopping and cleaning and what with her illness she herself only left the house to go for treatment. They had always lived in the same apartment on the ground floor thank God. She looked exactly like Mama and not at all like Papa, who had "gone on a trip" before she was born and had left behind only the apartment and a photo of himself you would swear it was Rudolph Valentino. Long ago she had worked at the Maternal Nursery School, not as a schoolmistress of course but in the office in the files. Later she had worked at the Paternal Insurance Company, isn't that an amusing coincidence, where she kept the files of work accidents. And then no she was in too much pain, she couldn't walk any more, her foot had become all stiff and here it was ten years already that she was living at home with Mama, who was in good health thank God.

The telephone rings. It's her doctor, who thought her appointment was for the next day. He confesses his perplexity with her case. Is she suffering from decalcification, from a form of sclerosis, from the effects of a childhood accident that had been poorly treated, or from the aftereffects of polio? He doesn't really believe in these possibilities but can't be sure. He had her take every possible and imaginable test, had sent her to a mass of specialists, but no one could make a convincing diagnosis.

I hang up, ask Mlle. O. to stand and take a few steps. She can't bend her left foot. She places, therefore, only the tip of the foot on the ground, never the heel. The other foot, turned severely toward the inside, is an accumulation of bunions and dead skin; the toes are deformed, tense, squashed against one another. Even with a cane, she walks with great difficulty.

I help her to lie down on the floor and to raise her legs to a right angle. It's not too difficult, even though the knees turn even more toward the inside. The adductor muscles, the "muscles of virginity," extending from the pubis along the inside of the thighs, are astonishingly stiff and maintain her legs tightly locked.

"At night, I have terrible cramps on the inside of my thigh. Often they wake me up in the middle of a dream. I always have the same dream."

I say nothing, wait for the rest.

"I dream that I'm falling."

Fine. I take her feet in my hands and ask her to close her legs even tighter. She cries out in pain, tries to free herself from my graps. The fronts of her thighs are in knots. I ask her to push the heel of her left foot toward the ceiling. Indignant, she says, "But that's the reason I came here. I can't do that." I offer to do it for her. The foot resists. I insist. A feeble movement. I insist again and the foot bends, supported only by the tips of my fingers. So her foot does move. So she could move it. I ask her to do it all by herself. Indignation again. She can't. Period.

I place her feet—the legs are still at a right angle to the floor—against the back of a chair and I start working on the back of her neck. She complains that her mouth feels dry. I ask her to turn her head from right to left. Protests and screams. When at last I lay down her legs, she moans uncontrollably. Her adductor muscles tremble in violent, spasmodic agitation. Shivering with cold, she murmurs, "You're tearing me to pieces. You're killing me." I cover her with a blanket and sit down next to her. I explain that her muscles can move, that they could make her foot bend and unbend but that she isn't sending them the appropriate orders.

"So it must be in my brain!" she said. "I must have a brain lesion!"

I ask her if she really believes that. Between her eyes, I can
see two deep creases. There's a new expression in her eyes. In a
voice that I don't recognize, she says, "No, I don't have a brain
lesion. But what I do have is in my head, isn't it?" I tell her that
head and body form a faithful and inseparable whole. I propose
that she come regularly and suggest that she could make a lot
of progress. She consents, then adds, "You'll see. I'll let you do
your work." I reply that in that case, nothing will change, that
it is up to her to do the work. She understands perfectly. She's
not at all as stupid as she'd like people to believe. She raised her
hand to her forehead, brought it down over her eyelids, her
cheek, her mouth. Behind her doll's mask, there was a woman
who'd waited fifty-nine years to begin to have a face. And her
body? How long was she going to wait before discovering that
she had a woman's body?

After she leaves, I feel nervous, tense, trapped by my sadness.
Françoise Mézières says that it's never too late to become aware
of your body, to discover your courage, your combativity, your
vital strength. But as I think of Mlle. O., of that long death
which has lasted all her life, I tell myself that it's also true that
it's never too early to become afraid of your body, and that that
fear is paralyzing, suicidal.

Fear of the body . . . fear of words . . . sometimes they're
inseparable. A person who has only fragmentary and fugitive
awareness of his body, who doesn't know it from within, needs
to stick a label on the wrapping. The word he thinks he must
use to define himself is often precisely the word he fears most.
"Pervert" and "homosexual" are two words that are dreaded by
many men and women who look for their "identity" at the same
time as they fear to find their undoing in them.

But the person who has resuscitated the dead zones of his
body, who knows or at least suspects the multiplicity of his desires and the richness of his ways of acting and reacting, can no
longer accept dictionary definitions. He discovers that definitions,

that nosography, are not appropriate to the new experience of his body: they can only keep it within the limits of his prior experience, define it in relation to what he has not dared to live until then.

Instead of telling himself the story of his life all his life long—of thinking and thus of being solely through the intermediary of words—he finally takes the time to listen to the subtle and varied messages of his body. He discovers that his body is himself and that he goes further, that he is richer and deeper than words. He discovers that he can stop the continuous monologue that is his thinking process and have proof of his existence through his sensations. It is then that he discovers a new language, a language of love that 'is absolutely personal and whose sole source of reference is his own body. In the multiplicity of his possibilities, of his desires, he discovers the multiplicity of his sexuality, his sexualities. Hetero–homo–bi—it is sexuality, the fact of his sexuality that counts, the fact of his fulfilled body.

Having become the vehicle of his imagination, his body, using as a departure point its own reality, can at last metamorphose itself in accordance with his desires and the desires of the other person. To metamorphose himself no longer means to deny himself, to hide himself, but to be all the possibilities of himself. A person who knows his body refuses only what's false to him, what he doesn't live in his body. Having freed himself from definitions, from repressions, from interdictions, he can know at last authentic sexual freedom.

8

The
Hospitable House

To take the risk of awakening your most painful archaic experiences and the dead zones they left as traces . . . to take the responsibility for the state of your body . . . to take cognizance of your body little by little until you feel that your life itself has "body" . . . "To take," yes, certainly. But afterward? Once you've been able to take, mustn't you become able to give?

Taking the responsibility for your life means assuming the cost of your maturity. (After a certain age we're responsible for our face, but also for our body.) But maturity is also being able to assume your responsibilities toward others. Toward your children if you are a parent. Toward your students if you are a teacher. Toward your patients if you are a doctor, a nurse, or a psychoanalyst.

I've often had the opportunity to see for myself how one person, by awakening his body, by gradually becoming more available to himself, modified the behavior of those who were called upon to "answer" his body language. Several men and women I treated were astonished to see their sexual partners magically blossom or rejuvenate as they themselves slowly discovered their own bodies. If they didn't immediately see the relationship between their own progress and the changes they discovered in their lovers, perhaps that's because it's hard to understand how we are lived or even that we are lived by another if, over the years, we haven't felt ourselves living.

Exactly what does happen when you become aware of your body? Sexually, the body which has been a façade gains in depth, assumes its third dimension to become a real house that's lived in at last and in which, potentially, two can live. Feeling stable, less vulnerable, you dare to let yourself be discovered by another. Available at last to your own sensations, you acquire a new sense of the other person. You discover his body, all the diversity of its expression, its emotions, its desires. Knowing what you feel, you can better imagine what another is feeling; your experience of your body brings you closer to his.

Finally in contact with himself, the person who has become aware of his body establishes new contact with those who are supposed to be "close" to him, but who had really been held at a distance. Sometimes, however, the other person refuses to allow himself to be approached. The story of Mme. G., who had been in one of my groups for several months and had made considerable progress, illustrates this situation well.

Forty years old, she had been married for more than twenty years to a man who could have been her twin brother. Prim, proper, perched on long, thin legs, they always made me think of a couple of grasshoppers. One day Mme. G. stopped making progress. She stayed at the same point for weeks. I wasn't concerned. I knew that students often pause at a landing before going on to their destination. But in the house of Mme. G.'s body, it wasn't a landing that kept her from continuing, but a door that had been closed. By her husband. "He doesn't want me to come here," she told me one day. "He says that working on the body is just egocentrism, narcissism. He even said . . ." I wait, say nothing. "That it's onanism," she whispered. I understood the gravity of the conflict when Mme. G. informed me that she'd be obliged to leave the group.

She who had just begun fleetingly to glimpse the depths of her life, would now never explore them. Not because she'd become afraid of her body, but because her husband had become afraid. Her way of living her body must have already modified her way of seeing him and perhaps of "receiving" him. So he protected himself with "isms." He accused her of being concerned only with herself when in fact the work she was doing on her body concerned him very directly, too directly.

Words lipped but not lived, words dropped condescendingly to those we speak down to, "isms" are often used by people who try to rule others' lives without putting their own on the line. When I learned that her husband taught children the same age as my own, my irritation turned to anger. Doesn't being a teacher mean that first of all we know a certain number of things about ourselves? When we present ourselves to a group of students, we consent not only to be heard but also to be seen, sensed, even touched. It is our body that we present and all that our body reveals about our life. If we consider our students more than just machines for recording our words, then our work can only be achieved body to body. (Why do we persist in calling a conversation between two people a "tête-à-tête" rather than a "corps-à-corps"?) Isn't the teaching body first of all the body of each teacher? The knowledge that a teacher proposes to his students is what he has learned about himself through reflection, of course, but also and simultaneously through the experience of his body. If a teacher isn't aware of his bodily presence in a classroom, today's students are often ready to let him know that they're not present just to take notes, but to take from him what he has brought to maturity within himself, the fruits of his experience. Isn't the body of a teacher a kind of tree of knowledge?

But what could be taken from a man who wanted to remain

ignorant of his own body, his wife's, and undoubtedly his students'? That man could offer his students only words—only "isms."

Sometimes a parent offers little more to his child. In any case, he doesn't offer him his body. He touches him with his fingertips, never caresses or envelopes him, kisses him only ceremoniously and at predetermined moments. When he finds that his child isn't developing normally, he's often ready to consult an army of specialists to find out why, never suspecting that there's only one pertinent question and he must ask it of himself. Let's take the example of Mme. D., whom I had been treating for several weeks for "scapulohumeral periarthritis." The extreme stiffness of this massively proportioned woman could also have caused her pain in the lower back, hips, and knees. One day she informed me that she wanted to show me her daughter. I agreed. When? "She's here now, in the entrance hall." My entrance hall is tiny, but I hadn't noticed a child there.

"Sylvie!"

Sylvie comes in, grazing the walls, and slips behind her mother, who, seated before me in the office, starts talking as though Sylvie weren't there.

"She isn't growing," she says in an accusing tone. "Four feet six isn't enough for a twelve-year-old. The pediatrician says that she's normal, but I . . ."

Sylvie has turned toward the bookshelves. I can barely see her face in profile. Her body is hidden by her mother's.

"From the day she was born until she was one month old, she never stopped crying. It was impossible to live with. So I gave her to a wet nurse in the country. When I took her back, she started to have terrible tantrums."

I'm not listening to her any more. I'm trying to see Sylvie's body. She's swaying from one foot to the other, stiff and regular as a pendulum. I see stuck-out shoulder blades, a neck that's hidden in the shoulders, a young, confused body, twisted like the stem of a plant that someone insists on turning toward the shade. I don't see any deformation that would justify an official label. It seems to me that the problem to be treated urgently is elsewhere. I tell that to Mme. D. She seems displeased. Either with my conclusion or with the fact that I interrupted her.

"Sylvie," she says without looking at her daughter, "wait for Mother outside." Sylvie makes a big circle around us and leaves before I can see her face.

I would like to tell Mme. D. that a child who's brought to "do physical therapy" is rarely motivated. He is there at his parents' or his doctor's command. The practitioner can always try to win him over, to explain to him what's wrong and why, to persuade him to "cooperate." But to what avail? His body has its reasons for growing twisted that the practitioner cannot know. I'm reminded of a famous laboratory experiment with two groups of guinea pigs fed in the same way and on the same schedule. However, only the subjects of the second group were, in addition, petted. And it is these animals who became by far the most vigorous, the most lively, the most resistent to infection. But I can't see how putting my thoughts into words can help Mme. D. She must have already heard and read thousands of words and look where it has gotten her. So in silence we start to work on her body again.

We worked together for over a year. Little by little the pains in her shoulder went away; her relapses occurred less and less frequently. The movement of her arm and her hands became less brusque. She started by granting short "leaves" to her military gait, then abandoned it altogether. The severe expression on her face became subtly modified, and sometimes she seemed quite reflective, grave. When she smiled, she used not only the corners of her lips, as she had before, but her cheeks, her eyes, her forehead.

After the last session before summer vacation, I accompanied her to the door. Two people were waiting in the entrance hall—

my next patient and a girl I didn't recognize. Mme. D. slipped her arm around the shoulders of the child, who stiffened a little, then let herself be enveloped. "It's her. It's my Sylvie," said Mme. D.

The child had grown more than four inches! She was well proportioned and held her head gracefully. She had a frank, intelligent, and, of course, slightly distrustful look. She passed in front of her mother, who whispered to me as she went out, "It all worked out. It's 'puberty,' I think."

Perhaps. But I think that Sylvie's progress was also the repercussion of the progress of her mother, who had finally consented to live in her womanly, motherly body.

Recently a sixty-five-year-old woman came to me with a major deformation of the spinal column, the result of a car accident in her youth. She had suffered every day for years. She told me that she was a doctor. But for the last two years her own pain had made her nearly an invalid and she no longer practiced.

While I was treating her, she asked me if I myself had ever known physical suffering. Her question disconcerted me completely.

"No, never," I said. Then, suddenly ashamed of myself: "Yes, once, a lumbago, but not very . . ."

She came to my rescue.

"I would have thought that you had suffered because you seem attentive to what the other person is feeling."

She explained to me that her own suffering had always made her sensitive to her patients' suffering. In her opinion, only those who have known suffering ought to be doctors.

I replied that sensitivity to others' bodies could be learned in other ways than through pain, but that it was certainly true that this sensitivity was lacking in a great number of doctors. Instead of calling them heartless, it might be more accurate to say that they are bodiless. Scarcely living in their own bodies, perceiving themselves as heads or hands, they can't consider their patients as whole beings. For these doctors, patients are ailments. Interested only in the ailment without taking into account the human being who is ailing, they reduce their patients to "nonpersons" before whom they often discuss the "case" in the most brutal terms. And then there are those doctors who are afraid of their own body, or are so prudishly embarrassed by it that they become incompetent when called upon to examine their patients thoroughly.

For some time now medical students have been required to take courses in psychology. That's certainly a step in the right direction. But wouldn't it be better still if *before* opting for medicine, candidates took "courses" in body awareness? Instead of being limited to the study of anatomical drawings and to dissections of cadavers, their knowledge of the human body— of the human being in his totality—would be enriched through research done on their own person.

By becoming conscious of their muscular "blocks" and by looking for their origins, how many of these young students would better understand their real reasons for having chosen medicine? How many who had believed they had a true vocation would discover that in choosing medicine they had simply yielded once again to parental and social pressures and that their body was rebelling, was rejecting a future that they didn't really want at all? How many would understand that they had chosen roles of responsibility and authority exactly because they didn't dare assume the responsibility for their own autonomy?

"Ever since I started rolling on the floor with my patients, I feel much better," an American psychoanalyst told me one day.

That's something already. But if she had become aware of her body *before* having launched into "touch therapy"—very fashionable that year—her patients would have been able to have taken more from her, been more in touch with her and with themselves. Or perhaps she would have discovered that if she had just naturally allowed herself to touch her patients with spontaneous and authentic gestures, she wouldn't have needed such violent demonstrations to prove her reality to them and for them to express theirs.

It is true that in psychiatric hospitals they are beginning to grant importance to the corporal behavior of the mentally ill. But they are still very far from recognizing the importance of the corporal behavior of those who treat them.

For example, they use "mothering" techniques. They bottle-feed the patient. They wrap him in moist sheets in the hope of awakening his sensations. But in approaching a patient's body through objects, in offering him palpable symbols, in acting "as if" and expecting him to play the game, isn't the patient's body, too, reduced to a manipulatable object? Isn't it most important for the person who offers the objects to be not just an intermediary instrument himself, but a real person living in a real body? The authenticity, the warmth, of the practitioner's gestures can do much more good, it seems to me, than the artificial techniques that are supposed to be "humanized."

In *Self and Others*, the anti-psychiatrist Ronald Laing tells the story of a schizophrenic woman to whom a nurse gave a cup of tea. "This is the first time in my life that anyone has ever given me a cup of tea," the patient told her.

Since this scene took place in Great Britain where drinking tea is a daily ritual, it seemed impossible that the patient was telling the truth. But she was. Laing explains that her extreme sensitivity about being recognized or not recognized as a human being, as a human body, allowed her to express a simple and profound truth: "It is not so easy for one person to give another a cup of tea. If a lady gives me a cup of tea, she might be showing off her teapot, or her tea-set; she might be trying to put me in a good mood in order to get something out of me; she may be trying to get me to like her; she may be wanting me as an ally for her own purposes against others. She might pour tea from a teapot into a cup and shove out her hand with cup and saucer in it, whereupon I am expected to grab them within the two seconds before they will become a dead weight. The action could be a mechanical one in which there is no recognition of *me* in it. A cup of tea could be handed me without *me* being *given* a *cup* of *tea*."*

To be there, behind the cup of tea . . . to be there, in our body, for ourself and for others . . . to live in our body . . . But, first of all, we must admit to ourselves that we have a body, that we are a body. And that being a body is our only objective and concrete truth.

Thought, sentiment, reasoning—of course we are that too and even more. But often we are all these things only because we say that we are. We content ourselves with words—treacherous, contradictory, fleeting—to tell us about ourselves, to invent ourselves. But it is essential for us to feel within our bodies who we are, that we are. Be a body first of all. Be a body at last. Be.

* R. D. Laing, *Self and Others* (New York: Pantheon Books, 1961), pp. 88–89.

Postscript

Is this a didactic book? A manual? Yes. But just a little. I'd call it a utopian book that points to a road that can take you toward yourself.

Perhaps it was necessary to write this book, to try to tell my own story and to grasp the essential of others', to understand just how difficult it is to become aware. And to understand what courage is needed, if not to start working toward awareness, at least not to abandon the work midway, or when we discover that we are our goal as well as our greatest obstacle. In persisting, we realize that we are going against the current: the more we advance, the closer we get to the beginning. Our body seeks its sources, its reasons for having become what it is. Through the body, our whole being learns that evolving means going from beginning to beginning.

In the introduction to this book, I made a list of results that those who become aware of their bodies could expect. It was so satisfying to enumerate, to promise; it was as though the good were already done. In this postscript, written one year later, it's with a new humility that I add: let's dare to begin.

Preliminaries

Here is the description of some Preliminaries, those movements I talked about earlier. It's best to be wary of them. No, they can do absolutely no harm to your body. The danger lies in granting them an authority to which you submit yourself, because you expect them to give you a new awareness of your body. But body awareness cannot be given. No movement, no method, can do that. Body awareness can only be taken. And only by those who allow themselves to.

But how do you go about becoming aware of your body? First of all, don't start out determined to get an "A+" in Preliminaries. It's much more important to fail—and to discover in that way what your body can't do yet, what it doesn't dare to do, what it has forgotten. "Taking" body awareness is a question of taking your time—as you'd take your pulse. It's not just a question of going slowly, but of going at *your* slowness, at the rhythm that you alone can feel from within your body.

This written description of the Preliminaries can give you only a slight idea. It is just a sketch of the vibrant improvisation that a real lesson given by an experienced teacher should be. Every lesson is "made to order" according to the student's needs and takes into account his prior experience and his receptiveness. The teacher's voice, the tone and rhythm of his words, the presence or absence of other students, the simultaneously neutral and familiar room where the class takes place, its special atmosphere—each element contributes to bringing the student closer to his body.

An "inspired" improvisation, a successful lesson, nonetheless has a classical structure similar to that of a play or a detective story. There is a gradual development toward a climax followed by a brief period of adjustment to the new situation—and life goes on.

Since you're going to be working alone, I recommend that you start each session with the first Preliminary. This allows you to know where you're at and to feel what your body needs first. After the first Preliminary, do the one your body seems to call for. Don't try to do them all in a row. You get more out of doing just one if you do it attentively, at your own rhythm. You should know, however, that often a tense shoulder will relax if you work on your foot. It's not necessary to tackle the pain directly. But your own body will tell you all that and even more—if you'll allow yourself to listen to it.

1. Undo your clothing, everything that restrains your body. "Why no, my bra isn't too tight. I'm used to it," is a common remark, when actually the body is furrowed with deep marks.

Lie down flat on your back on the floor. Arms alongside the body, palms turned toward the ceiling, feet falling where they will. Let the silence settle in. It will be easier if you close your eyes. Maybe you're not very comfortable. Be patient. Don't change anything. Just observe. What are the points of contact between your body and the floor? Do you feel yourself against the floor, and how do you feel:

Your heels? One heel with respect to the other?

Your calves? Buttocks? Pelvic bones? Sacrum?

Your back? How many vertebrae are touching the floor?

Your shoulder blades? With respect to the spinal column? With respect to one another?

Your shoulders? Do you feel their distance with respect to the ground?

Your head? Do you feel its weight? Its point of contact with the floor?

Pay attention to your jaws. If they're clenched, try to unclench them. Let your tongue spread out. Let it occupy all its space in the mouth. Fine. This is the beginning of the work.

2. This Preliminary uses the foot as the point of departure. You need a small foam rubber ball the size of a tangerine. Stand up and place the ball under your right foot. Gently massage the bottom of your foot with the ball. Massage underneath your toes, the ball of your foot, the middle of the foot. Keep the toes horizontal, extended straight out from the foot. Do not curl them up toward the ceiling. Put your weight on your right foot. In small circles, gently and methodically, continue to massage the entire foot: the heel, the inner edge and the outer edge. Feel that the skin and the muscles of your foot welcome the ball. It is possible that certain areas might be painful. Don't assault them brutally. Gently massage the periphery. Come back only when the foot permits it.

Afterward you can stretch out and compare the two halves of your body. Or, if you prefer, bend forward and try to feel if you come down with greater ease on one side than the other. Then "do" the other foot.

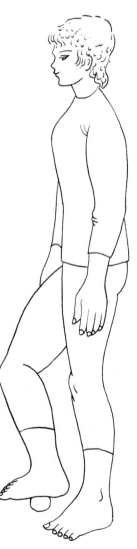

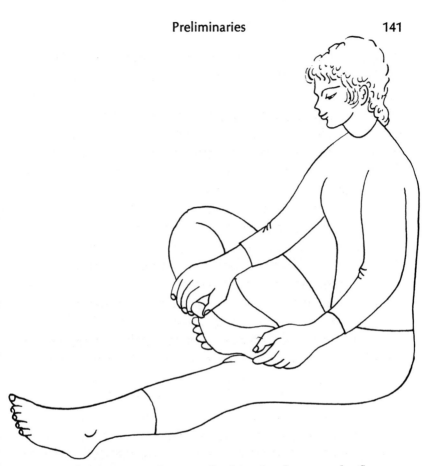

3. This Preliminary also uses the foot. Sit down on the floor, as comfortably as possible. Place the right foot on the extended left leg. Take the big toe of the right foot in one hand while holding the foot with the other hand. Pull gently on the big toe while turning it slightly, as though to unscrew it. Then turn it back to where it was. Do the same thing with the second toe, the third, the fourth, the fifth. Don't hurry. Pull and turn from the spot where the toe begins. Each one corresponds to a different zone of the spinal column.

Now, with the right leg flexed, place the raised right foot in front of you, but keep the toes in the line of the foot. They should not be turned up. (Your left leg is still stretched out.)

Take the big toe of your right foot in one hand. Take the four other toes in the other hand. Gently separate the big toe from the others.

A right angle should appear between the first and the second toe. Above all, don't force. You can take weeks to arrive at this stage. Toes are more accustomed to overlapping one another when forced into shoes than to being separated in this way. Now see if a right angle appears in the gap between the second and third toes, the third and fourth, the fourth and fifth.

Take your time and lie down on your back, legs extended. Compare how the two halves of the body are resting on the floor: the heels, the calves, the buttocks, the back, the shoulders. With a little experience, you will even be able to compare the two halves of your face. I'm not going to tell you what you will discover. But it will be a pleasant surprise.

If you feel the need to, you can "do" the left foot immediately afterward. Or else you can continue to work on the right foot. Place the palm of your left hand against the sole of your right foot and cross the fingers of your hand with the toes of your foot. In other words, pass your fingers between your toes. Be careful to pass one finger between each toe and not to take two toes together. Push gently down to the spot where the toe begins. It might hurt in the beginning. Now bend the front of the foot toward the ball of your foot until you can see the metatarsophalangeal joints. Stand up slowly. Compare your feet, placed side by side. Take a few steps. Which is your "real" foot?

4. This Preliminary is sometimes called "the hammock." Mme. Ehrenfried recommends it for women who have painful menstrual periods, but everyone can derive benefits from it. You need a fairly soft ball, the size of a large grapefruit. Lie down on your back, legs bent, feet flat on the floor and separated a little (to the width of the hips). Separate your knees a little, too. Try to release any useless tension: in your legs, especially the

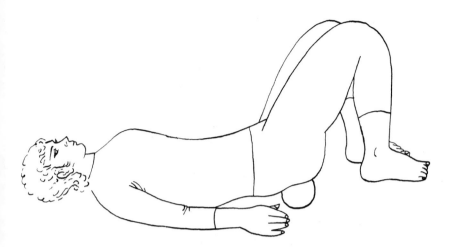

adductor muscles on the inside of your thighs, in your jaws, in your shoulders. Place the ball under the sacrum and the coccyx. And then don't do anything else; that's the hardest part.

Let your back come down slowly, close to the ground, and take on the shape of a hammock. Your stomach is supple. Your navel is falling toward the spinal column. Buoyed up by the ball, your pubis is aimed toward the ceiling. Your waist is resting on the ground. That's all. But if the retractions of the spinal muscles are too severe, you might need several weeks to be able to do it. You can check to see if your stomach is supple by placing your hand on it. No sense in fidgeting to achieve results. Let things happen. Now remove the ball. Observe how the lower back settles against the floor.

5. This movement involves extending the legs. Lie flat on your back, legs flexed, feet on the ground, the back of the neck as long as possible, which is to say, chin pulled in toward the neck. Take the front part of your right foot in your right hand and gently try to unbend the right leg and point it toward the ceiling. It's

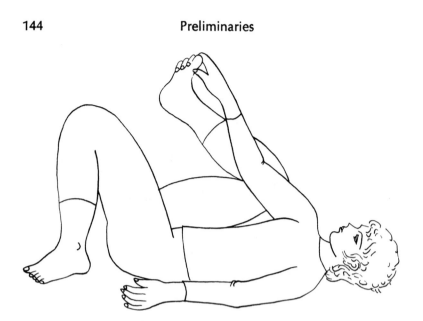

important to let the spinal column lie as flat as possible to eliminate all tension in the shoulders, and to feel that the right half
of the back is elongated. The best thing is to tell yourself that
you don't really want to straighten your leg out. It doesn't matter
whether you do it or not. Above all what you do want is to
coordinate the movement with your breathing. As though you
were breathing with your leg! When you exhale, you unbend
your leg and when you bring it back again, you inhale. The
exertion—for there is exertion—therefore takes place when you
exhale.

Patiently, slowly, deliberately, work on your right leg. Then
lie down completely. Compare the way in which the two legs
rest on the ground. Now stand up. Compare the way the two
sides of your body feel in relation to the floor. What difference is
there between the right leg and the left leg? How do you feel the
weight of the body on each foot?

Now lie flat on your back again, the legs flexed in the starting
position, and try to unfold both legs at the same time. Compare.
Don't stay wobbly; "do" the left side as well.

6. To work on your shoulders, sit down on a stool, your two feet flat on the ground. Your weight is distributed equally on the two ischia (pelvic bones which you can feel under your buttocks). Place your right hand on your left shoulder, directly against the skin. Not on the tip of the shoulder but right in the middle between the tip and where your neck begins. You have ample space to place your palm there. Grasp the trapezius (shoulder muscle at the side of the neck) in your whole hand. Be gentle but firm; the trapezii are often very contractured there. Let the left arm hang down. Then shrug the left shoulder. Tiny, light shrugs. As though you were testing the movement. Then turn the shoulder very slowly from front to back. Imagine that you are sketching perfect circles with the

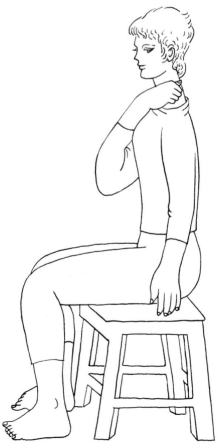

round tip of the shoulder. You want to do this while firmly holding the trapezius so that it will play as slight a role as possible in
the movement. One movement per breath will be enough. Avoid
having the left elbow follow the movement. The arm must really
hang loose.

Now let the shoulder go. Let the two arms hang down. Turn
the two shoulders together. You will feel right away which of
your shoulder is now "oiled."

7. To work on the neck, sit down on a stool and slowly turn
your head toward the left shoulder, then toward the right, and
try each time to look behind you. Grasp with your whole hand

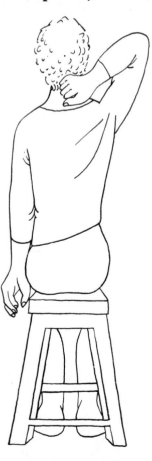

not only the skin but also the muscles of the back of your neck.
Try to unclench your jaws and relax the tongue. You're holding
yourself by the back of your neck, as you would hold a kitten.
Make very small nods with your head—"yes"—several times.
Your head is as relaxed as that of those little dolls whose heads
are attached by a spring. Then make little "no" movements.
Then draw tiny circles with the tip of your nose. Don't forget
to breathe. Now let go of your neck. Once again, look behind you
to the right and then to the left. Feel your new range of movement.

8. To work the shoulders, lie down on your right side, both
knees very flexed and resting on the floor, left knee resting *over*
the right knee. Your right arm is lying perpendicular to your
body. Your head, temple, and, if possible, right cheek are resting
on the floor.

It's important to settle yourself comfortably, as though you
wanted to go to sleep. Pay attention to your breathing at first.
Don't try to alter it. Then lift your left arm toward the ceiling,
elbow unbent, hand open.

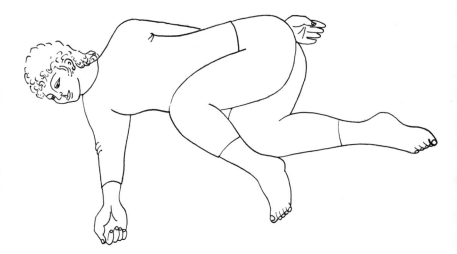

When you breathe in, slowly make your arm and shoulder go up toward the ceiling, then bring them down. Try to become aware of the movement of your shoulder blade, which you're making slide diagonally toward your waist as you come down and breathe out. Be aware also of the movement of your collarbone. You go up as you inhale. You come down as you exhale, quietly, through the nose, without forcing either the movement or the breathing. Do this about ten times.

Then let your arm fall behind you, close to the buttock. Your hand is loose, palm turned toward the ceiling, your forearm heavy, relaxed. Can you leave your head on the ground? Can you feel there's a lot of room between the ear and the shoulder? Proceed gently; don't force anything. Try to become aware of the exact spot where you feel restrained (in front of the shoulder? behind it? between the ear and shoulder?). Imagine that you're breathing in that very spot.

Then, on the next breath, just when you need to inhale, let the arm move away from the buttock, hand and forearm hanging behind. At the moment you exhale, stop the movement. Start it again when you inhale again. In this way, the arm traces a quarter circle backward. Very slowly. Do this in small stages and above all don't force the movement.

Gently bring the arm back near the hip. Stretch out on your back, legs flexed, and compare the two halves of your body: contact of the shoulders, the arms, the shoulder blades with the floor, the way you breathe on the side that has just exercised in relation to the other side, the feeling in the two halves of your face.

9. This Preliminary is a favorite of many of my students. It can have the same effects as a beauty facial. But it's less expensive and, in the long run, gives more convincing results. All you need is a ball about the size of an orange. Not too lightweight. An orange, actually, does the job very well.

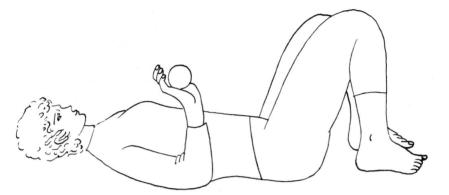

Stretch out flat on your back, legs flexed. The feet are placed neither too close nor too far from the buttocks so the waist can rest comfortably on the floor. The inside of the thighs is not contracted. The arms are parallel to the body, palms toward the floor. The ball is near the right hand. With your fingertips and without lifting your shoulder, elbow, or forearm, gently roll the ball parallel to your body toward your feet. Imagine that your arm is elastic. It is lying firmly on the ground. Slowly, with your fingertips, play at rolling the ball farther way, but without letting it escape you. Now take it in your palm and, pressing down on your elbow, lift up your hand (the palm is still turned toward the floor) and forearm. Slowly lift the ball toward the ceiling, without lifting your shoulder and elbow off the floor. You will feel the moment when the forearm become vertical. The ball is now resting in the hollow of your turned-up palm, thumb facing inward toward you. Your fingers spread out. Your palm becomes hollow; it becomes a nest for the ball. Try to feel the ball's contact, its weight in *the hollow* of your hand. Your fingers are no longer touching the ball. Be careful not to block your breathing. The air continues to circulate peacefully in the nostrils.

Gently place the ball near your body again. Lay both palms on the floor. Both arms. Take the time to compare their contact with the ground. You can also sit up and try to feel what has happened to the side of your face—your eye, the corner of your mouth, your cheekbone. You can verify your feelings in front of a mirror. But it's better to get used to being attentive to your feelings alone. Afterward, you can either do the left side right away or wait, if you want to become accustomed to feeling the difference.

10. This Preliminary will help you to rediscover your natural respiratory rhythm. Lie down flat on your back, legs flexed. Your feet are placed firmly on the floor, separated by the width of your hips. Your knees are slightly open. The insides of your thighs are relaxed. Place both hands on the front of your ribs, a little above the waist. Try to feel the movement of the ribs when you breathe, their direction when they separate. It's possible that you'll find very little movement—at first.

Now take a good hold of the skin under the edge of each side of your ribs and pull these two folds of skin straight toward the ceiling. When you inhale (through the nose), imagine that you're able to breathe directly from the interior of this fold of skin. When you exhale (through the nose), keep the skin

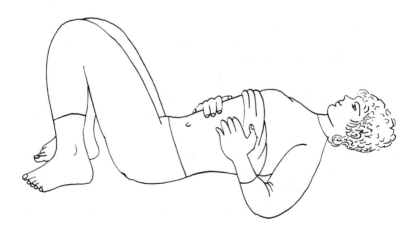

stretched upward. Never force your inward breathing. You should feel as if you're making more air go out than you've brought in. Breathe peacefully this way several times. Then release your skin.

Now take a good hold of the skin above your last ribs, behind and a little *below* your waist. Hold on to the two folds of skin and breathe peacefully just as you did before. Then release your skin.

Now observe the movement of your ribs. The rhythm of your breathing. Chances are that the movement is fuller and your breathing less rapid.

Mme. Ehrenfried recommends this movement particularly to insomniacs, and to those who have liver problems. It's also very good for the spinal column.

The diaphragm is the large muscle that "closes" the thorax. Where is it attached? Everyone knows vaguely. It's certain that it is attached to the periphery of the inside surface of the ribs in front. But in back, it's also attached to the spine: to the second, third, and fourth lumbar vertebrae. Each time you breathe, as the air enters and leaves the lungs, the diaphragm rises and descends on the inside of the body. Its movement alters the entire environment of the body. It gives the spinal muscles their freedom by not giving them a fixed point for contracting. You should also know that the diaphragm is situated just above the liver on the right side and above the spleen on the left. Its regular movement constitutes the "massage" which is necessary to these organs.

11. Here's a Preliminary that's hard to do alone. Try to have this passage read to you by someone. It should be read very slowly, with pauses between each sentence so that you can adapt yourself to what's being asked of you.

You are lying on the floor, preferably with your legs extended. But you can flex your knees, if that's better for you. Place your hands in the shape of a shell (fingers joined) over the eyes. Close your eyes. What do you see under your eyelids? Moving dots? Bright dots? Colors? Observe, then take away your hands. Keep your eyes closed. Imagine that they're sinking deeper into their sockets. Like pebbles that you'd let fall into a pond. Wait for the ripples to stop. Now you're interested in the right eyelid. You are making it very high and very wide. Like a big curtain over the eye. You're interested in the separation of the eyelids. In the way in which the upper and the lower lids touch. Do they simply touch? Or are they locked together? In your imagination, follow the rim of the two eyelids. Try to elongate the line that separates the eyelids, stretching it first toward the nose, then toward the temple.

Become interested in your right eyebrow. Follow it in your mind from the bridge of your nose to your temple. Imagine that you're pulling it toward the temple. Become interested in your tongue; let it get wider in your mouth. Your jaws aren't clenched. The tongue can even pass between the teeth. It takes up all the space in your mouth. You're interested in the outline of your jawbone on the right. Follow it from the tip of your chin to your right ear. You're interested in the inside of your cheek. Try to relax the muscles on the inside of the right cheek. You're interested in the right side of your upper lip. From the middle of the lip to the corner of the mouth. You're interested in the right side of your lower lip. Let it come up to meet your upper lip. Try to feel the air circulating in your right nostril, from the base of the nose to the right eyebrow. Imagine that you can breathe between your two eyes. Make a lot of room between your two eyebrows and breathe in that space. Put your hands back into a shell shape and cover your eyes. Observe colors or movement under your closed eyelids. Compare with your first impressions. You can sit up and try to see the difference. Now do the other side. Then thank the person who read you these directions. Be aware of the pitch of your voice. Has it changed?

12. For this Preliminary you need a foam rubber ball the size of an orange. You're lying flat on your back, legs flexed, attentive to the way in which your lower back, your waist, your shoulder blades touch the floor. Try to sense where the joints of the sacrum and the two bones (ilia) of the pelvis are located. You can use your hands to explore. Then let the pelvis rest on the floor again and place the ball under the joint on the right side. If you're not certain that you've found it, place the ball under the upper part of the buttock. Let the buttock press with all its weight on the ball. Let the left buttock press against the floor. Make sure that the waist is as close as possible to the floor. It's possible that the contact with the ball will be painful. Try to relax. Don't be on the defensive. Then, cautiously, raise your right knee toward your chest. Readjust the ball if necessary. Then place one hand on this knee and pull it toward you, little by little, without contracting the shoulders. Cautiously, straighten your left leg and continue to pull the right knee toward you as you become aware of the muscles along the inside of your thighs. Try to feel in what way they work together in this very slight movement. With the right hand, make the right knee draw small, well-rounded circles. Become aware of the circles that you feel being drawn at the same time by the part of the pelvic area that is pressing on the ball. Change the direction. Do several more circles. Then bend the left leg and gently put the right foot down on the floor. Take away the ball and

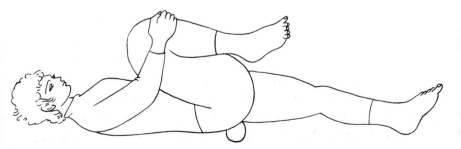

you'll immediately feel the difference in the pelvis. Turn on your side and then sit up. Now stand up slowly and walk around a little in the room. Pay attention to the (different?) way in which you feel your feet against the floor, to the way your right leg extends from the hip, to your right shoulder, to the right half of your face.

13. Do you remember those folded cardboard dolls they used to make? Joined at the top of the skull, one flap showed the front of the body, the other flap showed the back. Imagine that there's a line like that across the top of your skull, extending from ear to ear. Follow this line with your fingers. Then try to lift up the skin of the skull along the line. Pinch the skin between the fingers. You should be able to detach the skin from the skull at least a little. Pull a little on your hair if your skin won't move at all. Try to pull forward toward your face. All along the line, from ear to ear. As though you wanted to draw the skin of your skull forward, toward your cheekbones, toward your temples, toward your forehead. Try to arch the nape of your neck by bringing your chin close to the front of your neck, like a horse that arches its mane by lowering its nose. Imagine that you want to draw forward all the skin of your skull and your neck.

14. Gently grasp the skin between the base of your nose and your upper lip between your thumb and index finger. Pull downward gently. Your jaw is not clenched. Your tongue is wide in your mouth.

15. In ancient Chinese gymnastics, you are told to trace the contour of your ears with your thumb and index finger. Explore the pavilion (external part) of the ear between your fingers. Front and back. From where it's attached to your skull to the lobes. Explore the lobe. Front and back. Follow the antihelix, which separates the pavilion and the concha (and on which the spinal column is projected). From the antitragus above the lobe (where the cervical vertebrae are projected), to the top, under the fold of the edge of the pavilion (where the sacrum and coccyx are projected). Then gently explore the concha of your ear. Front and back. Finish by slowly massaging the entire surface of your ear.

Bibliography

Barthes, Roland. *Roland Barthes par Lui-Même*. Paris: Éditions du Seuil, 1975. Microcosme series.

Belotti, E. G. *Du Côté des Petites Filles*. Paris: Éditions des Femmes, 1974.

Borsarello, J. *Le Massage dans la Médicine Chinoise*. Paris: Maisonneuve, 1971.

Colette. *Les Vrilles de la Vigne*. Paris: J. Ferenczi & Fils, 1930, and Hachette, "Le Livre de Poche" series.

Davis, Flora. *Inside Intuition: What We Know About Nonverbal Communication*. New York: McGraw-Hill Book Co., 1973.

Ehrenfried, L. *De l'Éducation du Corps à l'Équilibre de l'Esprit*. Paris: Aubier Montaigne, 1967.

Feldenkrais, Moshe. *Awareness Through Movement: Health Exercises for Personal Growth*. New York: Harper & Row, 1972.

Freud, Sigmund. *Three Case Histories*. New York: Collier Books, 1963.

Greer, Germaine. *The Female Eunuch*. New York: McGraw-Hill Book Co., 1971.

Groddeck, Georg. *The Book of the It*. New York: Vintage Books, 1961.

Illich, Ivan D. *Celebration of Awareness*. New York: Doubleday & Co., Anchor Books, 1971.

Ingham, Eunice D. *Stories the Feet Can Tell: Stepping to Better Health*. Rochester, N.Y.: Eunice D. Ingham, 1959.

Janov, Arthur. *The Primal Scream: Primal Therapy, the Cure for Neurosis*. New York: G. P. Putnam's Sons, 1970.

Kafka, Franz. *The Penal Colony*. Translated by Willa Muir and Edwin Muir. New York: Schocken Books, 1948.

Laing, R. D. *Self and Others*. New York: Pantheon Books, 1961.

Lavier, J. *Points of Chinese Acupuncture*. Edited by Philip M. Chancellor. 2nd rev. ed. New York: Samuel Weiser, 1974.

Lowen, Alexander. *The Betrayal of the Body*. New York: Macmillan Co., 1966.

————. *The Language of the Body*. New York: Collier Books, 1971.

Mézières, Françoise. "Importance de la Statique Cervicale," *Cahiers de la Méthode Naturelle*, No. 51, 1972.

————. "Méthodes Orthopédiques" and "La Fonction du Sympathique," *Cahiers de la Méthode Naturelle*, Nos. 52–53, 1973.

————. "Les Pieds Plats," *Cahiers de la Méthode Naturelle*, No. 49, 1972.

————. "Le Réflexe Antalgique a Priori," *Cahiers de la Méthode Naturelle*, No. 44, 1970.

Michel-Wolfromm, Hélène. *Cette Chose-là*. Paris: Grasset, 1970.

Nogier, Paul. *Traité de l'Auriculothérapie*. Moulin les Metz: Maisonneuve, 1973.

Reich, Wilhelm. *Character Analysis*. Translated by Vincent R. Carfagno. New York: Farrar, Straus & Giroux, 1972.

————. *The Function of the Orgasm*. Translated by Theodore P. Wolfe. New York: Meridian Books, 1971.

————. *The Sexual Revolution*. Translated by Therese Pol. New York: Farrar, Straus & Giroux, 1974.

Sapir, M. *La Relaxation: Son Approche Psychanalytique*. Paris: Dunod, 1975.

Schilder, Paul. *Image and Appearance of the Human Body*. New York: International Universities Press, 1958.

Schultz, J. H. *Le Training Autogène*. Paris: Presses Universitaires de France, 1974.

About the Authors

Thérèse Bertherat practices the Mézières method of physical therapy and teaches "anti-gymnastics" in Paris. Her collaborator, Carol Bernstein, is an American copywriter.